PUBLIC HEALTH: PRACTICES, METHODS AND POLICIES

DIABETES MELLITUS

A MEDICAL HISTORY JOURNEY

PUBLIC HEALTH: PRACTICES, METHODS AND POLICIES

Series Editor: Joav Merrick, Medical Director, Health Services, Division for Intellectual and Developmental Disabilities, Ministry of Social Affairs and Social Services, Jerusalem, Israel

Environment and Public Health: Environmental Health, Law and International Perspectives
I. Leslie Rubin and Joav Merrick (Editors)
2014. ISBN: 978-1-63463-167-9 (Hardcover)

Tomorrow's Leaders: Service Leadership and Holistic Development in Chinese University Students
Daniel T.L. Shek, Andrew M.H. Siu and Joav Merrick (Editors)
2015. ISBN: 978-1-63321-880-2 (Hardcover)

Arbovirus: Public Health Experience from Zambia
Seter Siziya, Mazyanga L. Mazaba, Joav Merrick (Editors)
2015. ISBN: 978-1-63463-601-8 (Hardcover)

Health Issues in Diverse Cultures
Cecilia Obeng, Samuel Gyasi Obeng and Joav Merrick (Editors)
2015. ISBN: 978-1-63463-613-1 (Hardcover)

Public Health, Social Work and Health Inequalities
Bruce D. Friedman and Joav Merrick (Editors)
2015. ISBN: 978-1-63482-838-3 (Hardcover)

Environmental Health Disparities: Costs and Benefits of Breaking the Cycle
I. Leslie Rubin, and Joav Merrick (Editors)
2016. ISBN: 978-1-63484-211-2 (Hardcover)

Smoking and Adolescence: International Public Health Experiences
Mazyanga L. Mazaba, Seter Siziya, Joav Merrick (Editors)
2016. ISBN: 978-1-63484-311-9 (Hardcover)

Public Health: Some International Aspects
Joav Merrick (Editor)
2016. ISBN: 978-1-63484-612-7 (Hardcover)

Medical History: Some Perspectives
Donald E. Greydanus, and Joav Merrick (Editors)
2016. ISBN: 978-1-63484-747-6 (Hardcover)

Public Health: International Aspects on Environment and Health
I. Leslie Rubin and Joav Merrick (Editors)
2016. ISBN: 978-1-63484-834-3 (Hardcover)

Education in Hong Kong: Service Leadership for University Students
Daniel TL Shek, Cecilia Ma, Li Lin, and Joav Merrick (Editors)
2016. ISBN: 978-1-63484-928-9 (Hardcover)

Higher Education in Hong Kong: Nurturing Students to be Caring Service Leaders
Daniel TL Shek, Andrew MH Siu, Hildie Leung, and Joav Merrick (Editors)
2016. ISBN: 978-1-63484-980-7 (Hardcover)

Measles: Epidemiology and Control of Measles in the Gweru Urban District in Zimbabwe
Tawanda Marufu, Seter Siziya, Mazyanga L. Mazaba and Joav Merrick (Editors)
2016. ISBN: 978-1-63485-559-4 (Hardcover)

Diabetes Mellitus: A Medical History Journey
Donald E. Greydanus, and Joav Merrick (Editors)
2016. ISBN: 978-1-53610-094-5 (Softcover)

PUBLIC HEALTH: PRACTICES, METHODS AND POLICIES

DIABETES MELLITUS

A MEDICAL HISTORY JOURNEY

DONALD E. GREYDANUS
AND
JOAV MERRICK

New York

NOTICE TO THE READER

Additional color graphics may be available in the e-book version of this book.

Library of Congress Cataloging-in-Publication Data

ISBN: 978-1-53610-094-5

Published by Nova Science Publishers, Inc. † New York

CONTENTS

INTRODUCTION

Chapter 1

Trends in Child and Youth Diabetes

It is estimated that 86 million adult Americans have prediabetes and with that, a risk of developing T2DM (type 2 diabetes) within one in ten patients. About 29 million people have actual diabetes, most with T2DM. It was estimated in 2012 that about 208,000 people under the age of 20 have diabetes in the United States, but there is little data available on the prevalence of diabetes in the adolescent population. A recent study looking at 12-19 year olds from 2005-2014 found the prevalence of diabetes at 0.8%, with 28.5% undiagnosed and the prevalence of prediabetes 17.7%, more common among boys (22%) than girls (13.2%). With about 9% of the total US population having diabetes, this a public health issue of considerable proportion.

Introduction

Physical activity is important for a healthy lifestyle and quality of life. For example, parks can provide opportunities for physical activity for both children and adults in their neighborhood (1). A study in 20 neighborhood parks in Durham, North Carolina with 2,712 children and adolescents showed that the type of activity area and presence of other active children were positively associated with physical activity, while the presence of a parent was negatively associated (1). Results showed that physical activity of girls was more strongly affected by social effects (like other active children), whereas physical activity of boys was more strongly influenced by the availability of park facilities (1).

A study from Finland of 37,699 adults looked at childhood adverse psychosocial factors and adult neighborhood disadvantage to understand if there was a link to increased cardiovascular disease (2). They found that combined exposure to high childhood adversity and high adult disadvantage was associated with cardiovascular disease risk factors (hypertension, dyslipidemia, diabetes, obesity, smoking, heavy alcohol use and physical inactivity), while exposure to high childhood adversity or high adult neighborhood disadvantage alone was not significantly associated with cardiovascular disease (2).

Another study with 1,842 adults from Brazil looked at the local retail food environment and consumption of fruits and vegetables and sugar-sweetened beverages (3). They found that availability in neighbourhoods was associated with regular fruits and vegetables consumption, but regular fruits and vegetables consumption prevalence was significantly lower among lower-income individuals living in neighbourhoods with fewer supermarkets and fresh produce markets. A greater variety of sugar-sweetened beverages was associated with a 15 % increase in regular SSB consumption.

NEIGHBORHOODS

A recent (4) study used data from the Multi-Ethnic Study of Atherosclerosis (MESA), which involved more than 6,000 men and women from six communities in the United States (New York, Baltimore, Chicago, Los Angeles, Twin Cities and Winston Salem) to look at how neighborhood environments may influence the risk for developing type 2 diabetes mellitus (T2DM). They wanted to investigate long-term exposures to neighborhood physical and social environments, availability of healthy food and physical activity resources and levels of social cohesion and safety in relationship to T2DM. During a follow-up period of about ten years of adults aged 45-84 years at baseline 616 out of 5,124 participants (12.0%) developed T2DM and the study found a lower risk for developing T2DM associated with greater cumulative exposure to indicators of neighborhood healthy food and physical activity resources (4).

The studies above are just examples of recent research interest into the interrelation between neighborhood and the effects on health (5). This relationship is complex and also very hard to research, since it is multidisciplinary and multi agency with different community development policies, urban planning, zoning and transportation policies involved. In order to better understand the role of these environments and identify the most effective interventions in order to improve health will require partnerships between researchers, the neighborhood communities and policy makers.

DIABETES, CHILDREN AND YOUTH

There has been an increase in both T1DM (type 1 diabetes) and T2DM in children and youth (6, 7) and diabetes is no longer a rare disease in school-aged children. T1DM is still the leading cause of diabetes in children and accounts for about 5% of all diagnosed cases of diabetes (8). T2DM used to be mainly diagnosed in adults, but now more often seen in children 10 years and older (8) and apparently a result of more obesity and life style changes that has occured also in the pediatric population (8).

The American Diabetes Association and the American Academy of Pediatrics have therefore provided consensus statements and guidelines on both T1 and T2DM (9-12).

TRENDS IN PEDIATRIC AND ADOLESCENT DIABETES

It is estimated in 2012 that about 208,000 persons under the age of 20 years have diabetes (6, 8), but there is little data available on the prevalence of diabetes in for example the adolescent population (13).

A recent research letter in JAMA (13) examined data from the National Health and Nutrition Examination Survey (NHANES) from 2005 to 2014. This survey is representative of the civilian, non-institutionalized United States population, which both include in-person interviews and examinations in mobile centers (13). The authors used data collected from adolescents aged 12-19 years randomly selected to have blood glucose testing after fasting. In 2,606 adolescents they found that 62 had diabetes and 512 had prediabetes with the finding that among those with the disease, 20 had not even been diagnosed (13).

The prevalence of diabetes was therefore 0.8%, with 28.5% undiagnosed and the prevalence of prediabetes was 17.7%, more common among the boys (22%) than the girls (13.2%). These figures were much higher than previous estimates of diabetes prevalence among teenagers (0.34%) (13). Diabetes and pre-diabetes prevalences did not change over the time period in this study (13).

Black and Hispanic teenagers were more likely than white youth to have prediabetes and minority teenagers with diabetes were also more likely to be undiagnosed. Among black teenagers with diabetes, 49.9% did not know they had diabetes and 21% have prediabetes. Among Hispanic teenagers, 39.5% who had diabetes were unaware and 22.9% had prediabetes.

Conclusion

The United States CDC (Center for Disese Control and Prevention) estimated that 86 million adult Americans have prediabetes and therefore risk of developing T2DM (14), and 1 in 10 are unaware of their condition. About 29 million people have actual diabetes with most T2DM. With about 9% of the population having diabetes, we are talking about a public health issue of proportion.

References

[1] Bocarro JN, Floyd MF, Smith WR, Edwards MB, Schultz CL, Baran P, et al. Social and environmental factors related to boys' and girls' park-based physical activity. Prev Chronic Dis 2015 Jun 18;12:E97. Doi: 10.5888/pcd12.140532.

[2] Halonen JI, Stenholm S, Pentti J, Kawachi I, Subramanian SV, Kivimäki M, et al. Childhood psychosocial adversity and adult neighborhood disadvantage as predictors of cardiovascular disease: A cohort study. Circulation 2015 Jun 11. pii: CIRCULATIONAHA.115.015392. [Epub ahead of print].

[3] Duran AC, de Almeida SL, Latorre MD, Jaime PC. The role of the local retail food environment in fruit, vegetable and sugar-sweetened beverage consumption in Brazil. Public Health Nutr 2015 Jun 9:1-10. [Epub ahead of print].

[4] Christine PJ, Auchincloss AH, Bertoni AG, Carnethon MR, Sanchez BN, Moore K, et al. Longitudinal associations between neighborhood physical and social environments and incident type 2 diabetes mellitus: The Multi-Ethnic Study of Atherosclerosis (MESA). JAMA Intern Med 2015 Jun 29. Doi: 10.1001/jamainternmed.2015.2691. [Epub ahead of print].

[5] Diez-Roux AV. Neighborhoods and health: Where are we and were do we go from here? Rev Epidemiol Sante Publique 2007;55(1):13-21.

[6] Centers for Disease Control and Prevention. National diabetes statistics report: Estimates of diabetes and its burden in the United States, 2014. Atlanta, GA: US Department of Health and Human Services, 2014.

[7] Lipman TH, Chang Y, Murphy KM. The epidemiology of type 1 diabetes in children in Philadelphia 1990-1994: evidence of an epidemic. Diabetes Care 2002;25(11):1969-75.

[8] National Diabetes Education Program (NDEP). Oerview of diabetes in children and adolescents. Bethesda, MD: NIH, CDC, 2014.

[9] Silverstein J, Klingensmith G, Copeland K, et al. Care of children and adolescents with type 1 diabetes: a statement of the American Diabetes Association. Diabetes Care 2005;28(1):186-212.

[10] American Diabetes Association. Type 2 diabetes in children and adolescents. Diabetes Care 2000;23(3):381-9.

[11] Copeland KC, Silverstein J, Moore KR, Prazar GE, Raymer T, Shiffman RN, et al. Management of newly diagnosed type 2 diabetes mellitus (T2DM) in children and adolescents. Pediatrics 2013;131(2):364-82.

[12] American Diabetes Association. Standards of medical care in diabetes-2014. Diabetes Care 2014;37(Suppl 1):S14-80.

[13] Menke A, Casagrande S, Cowie CC. Prevalence of diabetes in adolescents age 12 to 19 years in the United States, 2005-2014. JAMA 2016; 316(3):344.

[14] Center for Disease Control and Prevention. National diabetes month-November 2015. MMWR 2015;65(45):1261.

SECTION ONE: DIABETES MELLITUS HISTORY

Chapter 2

A HISTORICAL JOURNEY OF DIABETES MELLITUS

This chapter provides a medical history synopsis behind the 21st century knowledge of diabetes mellitus, a disorder of terrifying tabescence known to ancient as well as modern homo sapiens. The term, diabetes, come from the Greek language and is attributed to Apollonius of Memphis in the 2nd century BC and Areteus of Capadocia (81-138 AD). There are many experts involved over thousands of years who helped unravel many of the mysteries of this disorder and these include Byzantine writers such as Greek physician Alexander Traillianus (Alexander of Tralles; 525-605 AD), Persian physician Rhazes (865-925), Islamic physician Avicenna (980-1037 AD), Jewish physician-scholar Moses Maimonides (1138-1204), British physician Thomas Willis (1621-1675), British physiologist-physician Matthew Dobson (1732-1784), the great French father of physiology Claude Bernard (1813-1878), French physician-biochemist-pharmacist Apollinaire Bouchardat (1806-1886), Lithuanian physician Oscar Minkowski (1858-1931), German physician Joseph Freiherr von Mering (1849-1908), and many others. Many millennia of wonder and research regarding diabetes mellitus was cyrstalized in the 20th century with the 1922 identification of insulin by the Toronto team (Sir Frederick Grant Banting [891-1941], Charles Herbert Best [1899-1978], John James Rickard (JJR) Macleod James [1876-1935] and James Bertram Collip [1892-1965]). The 20th century continued to improve the Toronto Group's work with the purification of as well as identification of the crystalline structure of insulin by biochemist John Jacob Abel (1857-1938), identification of two types of diabetes mellitus by Sir Harold Himsworth (1905-1993) in 1936, description of insulin's molecular structure by Frederick Sanger (1918-2013), development of NPH insulin by Hans Christian Hagedorn (1888-1971), the discovery of proinsulin by

Donald Frederick Steiner (1930-2014), and so much more as the 20th century faded into the 21st century. It is the story of the human mind steadfastly seeking to understand its world—a story worth telling again and again—a surrealistic story that has saved millions of lives from a premature death of misery in the 20th and now 21st century.

INTRODUCTION

The study of life began with the emergence of Homo sapiens over 200,000 years ago (1-6). Prior to the emergence of writing by the Sumerians in 3200 BC that emerged from earlier Neolithic writing, we can only guess at what ancient humans thought of a human disease with increased thirst and urination along with wasting of the body until death that we now call diabetes mellitus.

Rudimentary knowledge of medical conditions is traced to the Mesopotamia (3100 BC to 332 BC) that included Sumer and the Akkadian, Babylonian, and Assyrian empires in modern-day Iraq. The word, Mesopotamia, is Greek for “land between rivers” and indeed was between the Tigris and Euphrates rivers—major waterways of antiguity. Scholars who have looked at cuneiform clay tablets of this era identify references to descriptions reflective of urinary problems such as obstruction, urethritis (and urethral discharge), stones, and cysts (2-4).

Knowledge of ancient Egyptian medicine is known from such work reflected in the 1875 discovery by the German Egyptologist Georg Ebers (1837-1898) of what is called the Ebers Papyrus that dates to the reign of Amenophis I (second King of the 18th Dynasty) in 1536 BC (7-9). This document was over 20 meters in length and had 108 columns of text with a series of prescriptions organized by different diseases (7). The oldest known surgical document or text is the Edwin Smith Papyrus which was discovered in 1862 near Luxor, Egypt (8). Edwin Smith (1822-1906) was an American dealer and collector whose name was given to this papyrus.

Babylonian physicians based diagnoses on the appearance of urine (i.e., beet juice, wine, beer, paint, others) and therapy of renal or genitourinary conditions was with local remedies from local minerals or plants and blowing chemicals into the urethra. Alcohol served as an anesthetic. In their descriptions of urine these ancient physicians (1500 BC) commented on a disorder with “too great emptying of the urine” which is probably one of the earliest references to diabetes in the history of Western medicine; its treatment included sweet beer, wheat grains, and fruit (10).

Physicians were given considerable honor in ancient Israel and they were often priests from the line of Aaron.

> Honor the physician with the honor due him, [a] according to your need of him, for the Lord created him;
> for healing comes from the Most High, and he will receive a gift from the king.
> The skill of the physician lifts up his head, and in the presence of great men he is admired.
> The Lord created medicines from the earth, and a sensible man will not despise them.
> Was not water made sweet with a tree in order that his[b] power might be known?
> And he gave skill to men that he[c] might be glorified in his marvelous works.
> By them he heals and takes away pain;
> the pharmacist makes of them a compound.
> His works will never be finished; and from him health[d] is upon the face of the earth.
> (Old Testament Book, Ecclesiastes 38:1-8, 3rd century BC)

Ancient Physicians of India

This condition of excess urination was also identified by clinicians in India at approximately the same time as these ancient Egyptian physicians (1500 BC). These Hindus physicians in India described urine in the Ayur Veda that attracted insects (i.e., flies, ants) and gave diabetes its earliest name---madhumeha" ("honey urine") (10). One of the oldest medical traditions is the Indian Ayurvedic tradition---formed from the Vedic philosophies; two important texts were the Susruta Samhita and the Charaka Samhita (11).

Susruta of the Hindus (450 BC-380 BC), the father of medicine in India, recognized this condition in the 5th century BC (12, 13). In the spirit of 20th century Jacques Cousteau, these clinicians passed their understanding of science on to future clinicians to unravel the mysteries of this strange urination-wasting malady. Charaka and Susruta of India called it "Madhu Meha" in their Samhitas and the Susruta Samhita discusses increased urine (that was sweet), loss of weight, and other features associated later in the West with diabetes.

What is a scientist after all? It is a curious man looking through a keyhole, the keyhole of nature, trying to know what's going on (Jacques Cousteau: 1910-1997)

Ancient Greek physicians

Only by this historical route can many problems in medicine be approached profitably
(Sir William Osler: 1849-1919).

Western civilization's understanding of science is traced to the ancient Greek scholars and the first known Greek medical school was in Cnidus in 700 B.C. One of its early medical scholars was Alcmaeon of Croton (born around 510 BC) who helped to establish the principle of observing patients to understand disease (14). He was a student of the famous Ionian Greek philosopher and mathematician, Pythagoras (570 BC-490 BC). Though certainly influenced by ancient Egyptian medicine, these Greek physicians and scholars sought to move the knowledge of medicine further and indeed they did as they established the basis for modern Western medicine.

Table 1. Ancient physicians in the history of diabetes

Alcmaeon of Croton (born around 510 BC)
Susruta of the Hindus (450 BC-380 BC)
Thucydides (460 BC-400 BC)
Hippocrates of Kos (460-370 BCE),
Apollonius of Memphis (2nd century BCE)
Demetrius of Apamea (late first century BC)

One of the earlier movers in this direction was the Greek historian and political philosopher, Thucydides (460 BC-400 BC) of Athens who wrote the famous incunabulum, History of the Peloponnesian War, that detailed the 5th century BC war between the ancient enemies, Athens and Sparta. Thucydides is called the father of scientific history whose writings were based on verifiable data that did not include the effects of the Greek gods in the lives of human beings and rejected theories based on apotropaism. He noted that prayers were not effective in the treatment of medical disorders such as the plague. The age of scientific discovery was now born though based on the classic theory of humorism or the balance of the four classic humours (i.e., black bile, yellow bile, phlegm, and blood)---this Zeitgeist of ancient Greece persisted well after the Renaissance period into the 16th century!

Modern Western medicine traces its roots to the famous Greek physician, Hippocrates of Kos (460-370 BCE), who taught all future people of medicine to emphasize the patient and powers of observation, and not the disease itself or only rely on the leading of experience; the Hippocratic school speciously linked health and disease to four bodily humors (2,15). Its Corpus Hippocraticum was the beginning of modern Western medicine and is a link between ancient medicine and medicine of the 21st century. Hippocrates provided descriptions of the urine though not specifically with regard to diabetes:

> Bubbles appearing on the surface of the urine indicate disease of the kidneys and a prolonged illness.....colorless urine is bad.....the sudden appearance of blood in the urine indicates that a small renal vessel has burst… Corpus Hippocraticum (2)

However, the Hippocrates dictum of observing the patient encouraged others to make progress in the understanding of diabetes in the ancient world. An example is Apollonius of Memphis (Apollonius Memphites; Apollonius Stratonicus) who used the term "diabetes" (Greek διαβαίνειν [diabainein]—dia [through] + betes [to go]; Middle English diabete from the Medieval Latin diabetes--siphon). This Greek physician who was born in Egypt used this term to describe the condition "to pass through" in 230 BC (BCE) that was felt to be a kidney disease or form of "dropsy" and was treated with bloodletting and dehydration (10, 16). Caelius Aurelianus was a Greco-Roman physician and medical writer in the 5th century AD who wrote De morbis acutis et chronicus (Concerning Acute and Chronic Diseases) (17, 18). Caelius Aurelianus credits Apollonius of Memphis with using the term "diabetes."

Apollonius of Memphis was part of the school of anatomy in Alexandria, Egypt founded by Greek physicians Erasistratus (304 B -250 BC) and Herophilus (335 BC-280 BC). Herophilus of Chalcedon was the first anatomist and he described the anatomy of heart valves while Erasistratus further distinguished between veins and arteries in which one had a pulse (artery) and one (vein) did not based on vivisection work on the necks of pigs. Herophilus noted that arteries were thicker than veins and Erasistratus demonstrated the presence of semilunar valves. Based on the conclusions of the earlier philosophers (such as Plato and Aristotle) that the human body had no role after death, these Greek scientists at Alexandria began to dissect humans both dead and alive (i.e., vivisection).

Their work allowed physicians to conclude that the heart was not the center of sensations but was a pump to keep one alive. Erasistratus showed how blood was stopped from retrograde flow in normal conditions and that arteries were filled with air carrying “pneuma” or the “animal spirit (19).” He concluded that the blood flowed via vacuums. The removal of the anatomical location of the soul from the heart in ancient thought to the whole body and beyond was a process of many millennia that was stimulated by the knowledge of the heart as a pump and to explore complex human diseases (20, 21).

One of the students of Herophilus of Chalcedon was a Hellenistic physiologist in the late first century BC, Demetrius of Apamea (Asia minor). Demetrius of Apamea noted that increased urination (i.e., polyuria) was similar to a method called “racking” in which wine was siphoned between pots to remove dead yeast and encourage proper wine aging; he may have referred to this with the term, diabetes, or siphon (“passing-through”) (22). Thus, history often credits Demetrius of Apamea, a Hellenistic physiologist of the Herophilean school with the term, diabetes, and reflects the ancient view of polyuria as being caused by having ingested fluid pass through the person without changes as going through a tube.

THE FIRST AND SECOND CENTURIES AD

Scholars attribute the initial clinical description of diabetes to the writings of the first century Roman encyclopaedist, Aulus Cornelius Celsus (25 BC-50 AD) (10). Still surviving is his eight volume work, De medicina, which alerted his contemporaries and those to follow about this mysterious condition (23-25). One of these persons was Galen of Pergamos (Aelius Galenus or Claudius Galenus--AD 129 – c.200/c.216), father of modern and experimental Western medicine; he was a physician, surgeon, and philosopher (26-29). Galen was the son of a wealthy architect (Aelius Nicon) who shared a love of knowledge with his son and inspired him to become a foudroyant polymath for the ages.

Galen’s views on medicine and surgery were influential well into the Renaissance period in Europe. Galen felt that the strange disorder causing increased thirst and urination was a rare condition and named it diarrhea of the urine (diarrhea urinosa); the excessive thirst led to the term dipsakon (ardent thirst) (30). Galen did not agree with a theory contemporary with his times that this condition was a stomach ailment, but located it in the kidneys.

Table 2. Key physicians from the first two centuries in the history of diabetes

Aulus Cornelius Celsus (25 BC-50 AD)
Galen of Pergamos (Aelius Galenus or Claudius Galenus – AD 129 – c. 200/c. 216)
Rufus of Ephesus (80-150 AD)
Areteus of Capadocia (81-138 AD)
Chang Chung Ching (150-219 AD)

Rufus of Ephesus (80-150 AD) was a Greek physician and anatomist who wrote about diseases of the kidneys; he also developed the term, pancreas (pan for all and kreas for flesh) but did not connect diarrhea urinosa with the pancreas which he concluded was an organ in its place to guard posterior abdominal wall blood vessels (31, 32). This scholarly physician stressed the importance of precise nomenclature in anatomy and this influenced many of his colleagues as well as others who followed including Galen, Oribasius (see below), and many others. Parts of his treatises were preserved by medieval Arabic medical writers—particularly Rhazes (see below) (31).

Areteus of Capadocia (81-138 AD)

An important physician in the early history of diabetes is Arateus of Cappadocia (81-138 AD) from the late Hellenistic period; Cappadocia is in the eastern Asia Minor. He studied medicine in Alexandria, practiced in Rome, and provided important writings based on the Hippocratic Corpus and his own brilliant observations on many conditions including heart murmur, asthma, epilepsy, pneumonia, psychiatric conditions, diabetes and others (33-37). His eight volume book was written in Greek and was called "On the causes, symptoms, and cure of acute and chronic diseases (37)."

Arateus the Cappadocian provided further comprehensive descriptions of this condition and was the person who first distinguished between two types of diabetes—now called diabetes mellitus and diabetes insipidus (10, 35, 38-40). His description of this condition characterized by "melting away of flesh into urine" has resounded down the ages (35, 39). Diabetes was attributed to effects of cold and moisture reflecting the "pneumatic school" of thought (35, 41). His views were lost in later years until the first Latin version of his works were published in 1552 by Junius Paulus Crassus (Giunio Paolo Grassi) who died in 1575 (35, 42).

> Diabetes is a remarkable affliction, not very frequent among men…the patients never stop making water, but the flow is incessant, as if from the opening of aqueducts,,,the nature of the disease, then, is chronic,,,the patient is short-lived,….the death speedy….life is disgusting and painful….Hence the disease appears to me to have got the name diabetes as if from the Greek word…which signifies a siphon, because the fluid does not remain in the body, but uses the man's body as a ladder, whereby to leave it,,,,many parts of the flesh pass out along with the urine. (Arateus of Cappadocia (35))

Chang Chung Ching (150-219 AD)

In 200 AD Chang Chung Ching (Zhang Zhongjing [150 AD-219AD)]), a Han dynasty (206 BC-221 AD) physician called the Chinese Hippocrates, described the symptoms of diabetes mellitus and noted that the patient's urine was so sweet that dogs licked it (43-45). This urinary sweetness has been recorded in ancient India, China, and Greece and he was the first to test for diabetes with sweet urine (44). Chang Chung Ching is the best known of the ancient Chinese herbal physicians and wrote a book on herbal medication with two parts: Shang Han Lun and Chin Kuei Yao Lueh (Jin Gui Yao Lue). Many of these herbal remedies are still used in China and other parts of the world.

> We have come to understand that we are who we are is also who we were. (John Quincy Adams [1767-1848])

Byzantine writers (4th to 9th century AD)

Oribasius (325-403 AD) was a Greek physician living in the Oriental Roman Empire (Byzantium) who was born in Pergamum of Mysia (Western Turkey) and studied medicine at Alexandria under Zeno of Cyprus. He became the personal physician to the Roman emperor, Julian the Apostate (Flavius Claudius Iulianus Augustus: 331-363 AD) and was the leading physician as well as important medical historical of his time (46). Oribasius established

Byzantine nephrology and utilizing magnifying lenses, confirmed Erasistratus' concept of a connection (anastomosis which he called capillaries) between arteries and veins (47).

Table 3. Byzantine physicians/writers (4th to 9th Centuries AD) in the history of diabetes

Oribasius (325-403 AD)
Stephanus Alexandriensis (550 AD-622 AD)
Alexander Traillianus (Alexander of Tralles; 525-605 AD)
Aetius Amidenus (Aëtius of Amida---5th century AD)
Paul of Aegina: 625-690 AD)
Theophilus Protospatharius (7th century AD)
Stepanus of Athens (7th Century AD)
Leon of Pella (9th century AD)

He also identified circulation in the kidneys that including blood flow through the aorta's renal artery branch with venous return via the inferior vena cava's renal vein branch (47). Orbasius also provided descriptions of patients with diabetes as did other Byzantine writers from the fourth to the ninth century AD under the Graeco-Roman influence in medicine (see Table 3) (48). His writings included works of Galen and other medical writers of the ancient world that was found in 70 books with only 25 having survived in what has been called "Collectiones medicae" (49-52). Many of the ancient medical writers' works would have been lost to modern times except for the encyclopaedic contributions of Oribasius.

Observations were occurring in medicine in other countries as well. For example, Sushruta and Charaka were two Indian physicians from the 5th century who noted that persons with a thin physique developed symptoms of diabetes earlier than heavier individuals; these older patients lived longer than the thin ones with their symptoms---thus, recognizing two different types of disease later called type I diabetes mellitus and type 2 (10, 53).

Stephanus Alexandriensis (550 AD-622 AD)

Another Byzantine writer who commented on symptoms of diabetes was Stephanus Alexandriensis (550 AD-622 AD) who wrote about ancient physicians (i.e., Hippocrates as well as Galen) and taught at the University of

Constantinople that had been founded by the Byzantine Emperor Theodosius II (401-450 AD) in 425 AD (54-56). In addition to medicine Stephanus Alexandriensis also wrote about astronomy, philosophy and alchemy (alchemical work).

Alexander Traillianus (525-605 AD)

Alexander Traillianus (Alexander of Tralles; 525-605 AD) was a Greek physician born in Tralles in Lyia (now Turkey); his father (Stephen) was a physician and he had a well-known mathematician brother (Anthemios) who was the architect of the church Hagia Sophia in Constantinople (57-59). Alexander practice in Rome, Italy and wrote a number of treatises on medicine with the main one being the Therapeutics (Twelve Books on Medicine) while others included On Fevers, On Intestinal Worms, and others (57-61).

> I like to use every possible means in treating my patients.
> (Alexander Traillianus) (57)

Alexander Traillianus wrote about symptoms of diabetes and epilepsy while covering issues of craniofacial surgery as well (57, 62, 63). Persons with polyuria, polydipsia, and weight loss were felt to have a kidney disease—consistent with ideas of other Byzantine medical writers (48, 64). Some of his medical writing was translated into Latin around 700 AD and later to Arabic and Hebrew (57). A Greek text of some of his work was printed in Paris, France in 1548 and in Venice in 1570. Such translations allowed seminal Western concepts to be passed on to future generations despite the Dark Ages that began with the Fall of Rome in 476 AD.

> I have assembled from my rich experience of treatments of various diseases...although I am an old man and no longer able to exert myself greatly, I...wrote this book, after having collected my experiences from my many contacts with human diseases. And I know this will please many people who are not envious to look at the good reasoning of my medical theories and at the same time the brevity and clarity of the exposition. (Alexander of Trailles) (57)

Aetius Amidenus

An early to mid-6th century Byzantine physician who continued the Byzantine reflection of diabetes and kidney disease was Aetius Amidenus (Atius of Amida), though some scholars place him in the 5th century (48,64,65). He was a Greek born in Amida (now Diyarbakir, Turkey) and as was noted with many physicians of his era, studied medicine in Alexandria (66). Aetius Amidenus wrote on a variety of medical and surgical topics that included apoplexy, pelvic abscesses, pain relief (using opium), acne (one of earliest descriptions), ophthalmology, cranio-maxillofacial surgery, and others (65,67-75).

Paulus Aegineta (625-690 AD)

Paulus Aegineta (Paul of Aegina: 625-690 AD) was a 7th century Byzantine physician and writer who also wrote about symptoms of diabetes (48, 64). He concluded that diabetes was due to a disease of the kidneys and suggested a variety of treatments including blood removal (venesection), dark wine, myrtle, dates, juice from knotgrass, and lettuce. He was a Greek born on the island of Aegina, practiced surgery as well as gynecology in Alexandria and was a traveling physician whose best known book was called Epitome medicae libri septem (medical compendium in seven books), which was largely based on the writings of Galen as well as Oribasius and provided a summary of Western medicine at that time (48, 64, 76, 77). He was highly regarded by the Arab physicians of his day and into future centuries. His work set the stage for later development in surgery (including plastic surgery) with the sixth book that was devoted to surgery (78-81).

Li-Hsuan and Chen Chuan

During the same 7th century a Chinese physician, Li-Hsuan, also described diabetes noting that the patient with this condition had a tendency to develop skin infections (boils) and pneumonia; treatment included the avoidance of alcohol, starch and sex (10, 82). A Chinese colleague of Li-Hsuan, Chen Chuan also noted the sweetness of urine and named this disease Hsiao kho ping (for strong thirst, polydipsia, and polyuria with sweet tasting urine (46). Such urinary sweetness was not appreciated in the West until the observations of Oxford physician Thomas Willis (1621-1675) in 1674, as discussed later in this article (10, 39, 83). Li-Hsuan also commented on the sweetness of urine in these patents (84):

> This disease is due to weakness of the renal and urogenital system. In such cases the urine is always sweet. Many physicians do not recognize this symptom. The cereal foods of the farmers are the precursors of sweetness...the methods of making cakes and sweetmeats...mean that they all very soon turn to sweetness...It is the nature of the saline quality to be excreted. But since the renal and urogenital system at the reins [i.e., kidneys] is weak, it cannot distill the nutrient essentials, so that all is excreted as urine. Therefore the sweetness in the urine comes forth, and the latter does not acquire its normal color.

Theophilus Protospatharius

Another 7th century Byzantine physician and writer, though less known than Paul of Aegina, was Byzantine writer Theophilus Protospatharius who also commented on the symptoms of diabetes (48, 64). Byzantine management of his patients with diabetes included nutritional counseling, bloodletting, use of various herbs, herbal poultices for skin infections, and avoidance of diuretics (48). Theophilus Protospatharius is often identified as the Byzantine founder of urology with a written compiling of known information that was called De Urinis (85-88).

Contemporaries of Theophilus Protospatharius and Paulus Aegineta include Stepanus of Athens and Leon of Pella (9th century AD) who were Byzantine writers that also reflected on these difficult patients with polyuria, polydipsia, and weight loss before death (48, 66, 87, 89-94). Rhazea (865-925 AD) was an Arab writer who translated the Sanskrit into Arabic and discussed patients with symptoms reflective of diabetes (see below) (95).

> Stephanus' aim is to imbue his pupils with proper method and he contrasts the Hippocratic physician often with the 'idiot' physician, who through ignorance of the proper method commits error after error and who is led astray by a simplistic reliance on symptoms. But there are limits to a doctor's knowledge; only...a higher power knows everything or disposes health to every patient, and the workings of the heavens are not always revealed to the physician. Sometimes the responsibility for a patient's failure to recover can be

properly laid at the door of his doctor, but at other times chance and the vagaries of the patient himself must take the blame (90)

GOLDEN AGES OF ISLAMIC ERA: 9TH TO 12TH CENTURIES

The Fall of Rome in 476 AD led to a loss of medical knowledge in Europe though medicine was kept alive and advanced by brilliant Persian and Arab physicians in the 9th century and beyond (see Table 1) (47,96,97). As the Western world was hurled into the Dark Ages (476 BCE to 1000 BCE), they continued to study cardiology, nephrology, and other aspects of human health and disease (98-101). Persian-born physicians include Doctors Taberi, Magusi, and Razi (102).

Table 4. Arab/Persian Clinicians of the Golden Age of the Islamic Era (Partial List)

Ali at-Taberi (838-870 AD)
Ar-Razi (Rhazes:865-925 AD)
Ali ibn al-Abbas al-Magusi (Haly: died around 990 AD)
ibn al-Qasim al-Zahrawi (Abulcasis: 936-1013 AD)
ibn al-Haitam (Alhazen: 965-1040 AD)
ibn Sina (Avicenna: 980-1037 AD)
ibn Abi al-Ala Zuhr (Avenzor: 1091-1131 AD)
ibn Rushd (Averroes: 1126-1198 AD)
ibn al-Baitar (1197-1248 AD)
ibn al-Nafis (1213-1288 AD)

Rhazes

Rhazes (Abu Bakr Muhammad ibn Zakariyya al-Razi; 865-925), a musician turned physician, perhaps is the best known of the Persian physicians who is acclaimed as a father of pediatrics. Complications of diabetes were recognized by physicians in the 8th century and beyond (as Rhazes) that included vision damage, furuncles, and ulceration (46, 98).

Avicenna

Often acclaimed as the most influential Islamic physician/philosopher was Ibn Sina (Avicenna; Abou Ali al-Housayn ibn-Abdoullah ibn-Sina; 980-1037 AD) who wrote a medical encyclopedia called Cannon of Medicine (Qanun fil-tibb) and a work on cardiac drugs (98-100,103-106). His encyclopedic work, The Book of Healing, became well-known for eons (100,103). Avicenna was born in Bukhara (present-day Uzbekistan) and died in Hamadan; he was a prolific polymath in various fields including medicine, mathematics, physics, Islamic theology, astronomy, geology, and poetry. His father was a respected scholar and installed this love of scholarship in his son.

Avicenna refined Galen's theory of pulses and provided details on a number of drugs that effected the heart. He made mention of pericardial disease and prevention of cardiac diseases including the importance of a "healthy" diet for those with heart disease. In his book on drugs for heart disease there is mention of various drug treatments that came from mineral, vegetable, and animal sources (103, 104). He was the first to use a drug that eventually (i.e., modern times) was classified as a calcium channel drug (105). He described what was later called the Willis circle, capillary circulation, cardiac tamponade, hypertension, palpitation, stroke, hypersensitivity and its link with vasovagal syncope, and the connections of emotion with cardiac action (98,104).

He provided descriptions of diabetes as well as its complications such as sexual dysfunction (i.e., impotence), mental illness, furuncles, and gangrene (10, 46). Avicenna called this condition a water wheel (aldulab) as well as kidney diarrhea (zalkh el kuliah); he described diabetes with body wasting that was different from other causes of excess urination (106).

He treated this disorder with substances inducing vomiting and sweating, exercise (such as horseback riding), baths (lukewarm), "fragrant" wine, and avoidance of agents causing diuresis (107). The concept of exercise was to develop heat in the body to help with removal of bodily wastes and enhance digestion to prevent accumulation of toxins (109). Horseback riding was theorized to develop friction and improve polyuria. Some physicians in the 13th century treated diabetes with purgatives, astringents, and refrigerant remedies (107). Avicenna's work was influential for the next several centuries and even to the 21st century (108, 109-119).

In 1914 the highly-respected Sir William Osler write about the need to restore the tomb of Avicenna (111). Avicenna has been linked in medical writing to the description of a physician found in "Canterbury tales" by

Geoffrey Chaucer (1340-1400) as translated by the English literary scholar Nevill Josiah Aylmer Coghill (1852-1879):

> A Doctor too emerged as we proceeded;
> No one alive could talk as well as he did
> On points of medicine and of surgery,
> For, being grounded in astronomy,
> He watched his patient's favourable star...."

Ibn al-Nafis (1213-1288)

Ibn al-Nafis was an Arab physician who challenged the Galenic theory of circulation and did not agree with the belief in a porous interventricular septum (120,121). Ibn al-Nafis described the pulmonary circulation and wrote about pores between the pulmonary artery and vein that four centuries later were called pulmonary capillaries by Marcello Malpighi (120-123). Some have incorrectly noted that the 16th century European scientists discovered the pulmonary circulation but this distinction belongs to Ibn al-Nafis in the minds of some scholars (123-125). He was a famous ophthalmologist who also described the coronary circulation (124). Contributions of Inn al-Nafis sometimes are confused in the English speaking world since his and other works of physicians in the Islamic Golden Age of Medicine were published in Persian and/or Arabic.

> If I don't know that my work will not last up to ten thousand years after me, I would not write them. Ibn al-Nafis (123)

Moses Maimonides (1138-1204)

> A physician should begin with simple treatments trying to cure by diet before he administers drugs....Like unto a murderer is the physician who refuses to tender his assistance in time of necessary or who practices without due study of the ailment which he is treating. (Moses Maimonides, Commentary on the Mishnah) (126)

The great Jewish scholar, Moses Maimonides (1138-1204) was a prominent physician (as well as rabbi, philosopher, astronomer) born in

Cordova, Spain as the son of a noted Jewish rabbi (126-135). He lived in Spain as well as North Africa and eventually became the court physician to the sultan Saladin in Cairo, Egypt. He was called the Rambam based on his name of Rabbi Moses Ben Maimon; in the Arabic literature his name was Abu 'Imran Musa ben Maimun ibn' Abd Allah (126). He was a highly regarded scholar and physician as noted by this Arabic poem by Al-Sa'id ibn Surat al-Mulk:

> Galen's art healed only the body,
> But Abu "Imran's (Maimonides), the body and soul.
> With his wisdom he could heal all the sicknesses of ignorance.
> If the moon would submit to his art,
> He would deliver her of her spots at the time of full moon,
> Cure her of her periodic defects,
> And at the time of her conjunction save her from her waning (126)

Moses Maimonides provided much information on medicine such as nephrology that included expanding the understanding of urinalysis. For example, he gave descriptions of red urine (later identified by the eminent 19th century English physician, Richard Bright MD (1789-1858) as glomerulonephritis) and black urine (later identified as a sign of malaria) (98).

> You must accept the truth from whatever source it comes
> Maimonides

Moses Maimonides detailed various aspects of diabetes in patients including symptoms of acidosis (46,83). He provided many aphorisms about medicine that have sounded throughout the ages (133). As noted by Rodin, many have noted: "From Moses the lawgiver until Moses ben Maimon, there was none like Moses!" (126).

> The more perfect a person becomes in one of the sciences, the more cautious he grows, developing doubts, questions, and problems that are only partially solved; whereas one deficient in science will find it "easier to understand every difficulty. Moses Maimonides (1135-1204) (131)

RENAISSANCE ERA AND THE PANCREAS (1300/1400-1600 AD)

Abdel Latif el Baghdadi (Abd al-Latif al-Baghdadi; Muwaffaq al-Din Muhammad; Abd al-Latif ibn Yusuf al-Baghdadi; 1162-1231 AD) was an Arabic physician and historian who was also a prolific writer; he wrote a disquisition on diabetes that is still in existence (106). Diabetes was seen as a kidney disease and treatment included ways to ameliorate kidney strain with purgatives; other therapeutic measures included astringents and refrigerant modalities (107).

Table 5. Renaissance era physicians and the pancreas (1300/1400-1600) in the history of diabetes

Abdel Latif el Baghdadi (Abd al-Latif al-Baghdadi; Muwaffaq al-Din Muhammad) 1162-1231 AD)
Paracelsus (Theophrastus Bombastus von Hohenheim: 1493-1541)
Gerolamo (or Girolamo or Geronimo) Cardano (French: Jérôme Cardan; Latin: Hieronymus Cardanus) (1501-1576)

Parcelsus (1494-1541)

Paracelsus (Theophrastus Bombastus von Hohenheim: 1493-1541), a famous and colorful physician from Switzerland, wrote about proteinuria, hematuria, gout, and edema; his work was the forerunner of using specific gravity in urinalysis (2, 136).

Paracelsus (1494-1541) noted that a white residue was seen after the urine of a patient with diabetes evaporated; he thought this residue was salt and felt the etiology of diabetes was salt deposited in the kidneys (10, 136). History has also negatively identified Paracelsus as publically burning the treatises of Galen and Avicenna in 1527 in Basel, Switzerland that was part of the complex religious fervor of the 16th century Reformation Period in Europe.

Gerolamo Cardano (1501-1576)

Gerolamo (or Girolamo or Geronimo) Cardano (French: Jérôme Cardan; Latin: Hieronymus Cardanus) (1501-1576) was an Italian physician and mathematician who gained considerable fame for writing the first Latin work on algebra called Ars Magna (136). In his work as a physician, this brilliant Italian polyglot also looked at patients with diabetes, noted great differences as he measured their fluid intake/output, and concluded that these persons lose more water than they consume for reasons that eluded him as well as others in his century and beyond (137-141). He also became one of the infamous gamblers of the Renaissance (Scarani) (142).

Table 6. 17th and 18th century giants in the history of diabetes

Morgagni (Giovanni Battista Morgagni: 1682-1771)
Thomas Sydenham (1624-1689)
Thomas Willis (1621-1675)
Johann Conrada Brunner (1653-1727)
William Cullen MD (1710-1790)
Matthew Dobson (1732-1784)
John Rollo (died 1809)

PROGRESS IN THE 17TH AND 18TH CENTURIES

Table 6 lists physicians who were 17th and 18th century giants in diabetes. This includes the founder of pathological anatomy, Morgagni (Giovanni Battista Morgagni: 1682-1771), who described various renal disorders via autopsy (98,143). Diabetes in this era was felt to be a kidney diseases and Morgagni felt that the sweet taste of diabetic's urine was due to the fact that water and nutrients went unchanged into the urine (83). Though he started out with little fanfare, his acceptance by the great English philosopher, John Locke, and others led to his great acceptance by his peers (143).

Thomas Sydenham (1624-1689)

Thomas Sydenham was one of the most influential Western physicians of the 19th century who is often called the English Hippocrates (144-148). His fame was stimulated by his acceptance by the great English philosopher and physician John Locke (1632-1704) that led to widespread acclaim by his peers as his career unfolded (146). Sydenham theorized that diabetes was a systemic illness due to incomplete chyle digestion which also causes polyuria seen in these patients (147).

Thomas Willis (1621-1675)

Thomas Willis was a British (Oxford) physician and anatomist who was one of the greatest physicians of his time---he identified the circle of Willis, Willis's nerve and provided many other anatomical insights as the founder of modern neurology (46, 149-151). This giant of medicine separated diabetes in 1670 from other causes of polyuria by the sweet taste of the diabetic patient's urine and concluded the sweetness first was seen in the blood. He added the word "mellitus" for honey sweet and utilized this to differentiate diabetes mellitus from other conditions causing polyuria (46, 83, 152-154). Willis concluded that the sweetness was due to salts and acids (148, 155). He described diabetic neuropathy and concluded diabetes was a blood disorder though many of his peers viewed this condition as a kidney disorder; astringents were often used in its treatment (46, 107). Many clinicians in his day believed that diabetes was due to humoral changes and too much drinking of alcohol (107).

Willis' description of the autonomic nervous system provided him with insights in the contribution of emotion in disease. Thomas Willis insightfully speculated on the importance of emotion in diabetes in 1678; in his book, Pharmaceutice Rationalis, he theorized that prolonged sorrow ("sadness, long grief") was etiologically linked to diabetes along with strong wine (beer and cider) and nervous system juice (148, 156). His reflections led to future clinicians and researchers seeking to understand the impact of psychological issues in human disease, such as diabetes mellitus (157).

Johann Conrada Brunner (1653-1727)

Johann Conrada Brunner was a Swiss physician and anatomist who was a leading researcher of his era on the pancreas and duodenum (158). He performed experiments in dogs that included a subtotal pancreatectomy with reversible traumatic damage to the remaining pancreatic tissue (159, 160). After the canine surgery, Brunner noted in 1682: "....the animal made water very frequently and he was very thirsty, drinking largely of water in proportion to the discharge of urine (160)." Despite his successful surgery on 8 dogs that led to canine diabetes and his description of the induced symptoms (i.e., polydipsia, polyuria, polyphagia), Brunner did not associate this with diabetes and thus, the link of the pancreas with diabetes waited for conclusions of research in the late 19th century as discussed later (159-161). This is an example of some "near-misses" in understanding diabetes mellitus seen throughout medical history.

Matthew Dobson (1732-1784)

Matthew Dobson was a British (Liverpool) physiologist and physician who revealed in his 1776 work, Experiments and Observations on the urine in diabetics, that evaporation of urine of diabetic patients produced a residue that was a crystalline material with the taste of brown sugar (46, 162, 163). He noted that this material "was granulated and broke easily between the fingers; it smelled sweet like brown sugar, neither could it be distinguished from sugar, except that the sweetness left a slight sense of coolness on the palate" (162).

This process involved boiling the urine to dryness and he noted that the urinary sugar concentration was increased (163). He concluded that the urinary sugar first appeared in the blood and then in the urine; thus, he identified hyperglycemia and suggested that diabetes was a systemic disease and not a kidney disease that require special diets for treatment (10, 83, 136, 163, 164). Matthew Dobson noted that: "….that this substance had previously existed in the serum rather than being formed in the kidneys….."this idea of the disease explains its emaciating effects from so large a proportion of the alimentary matter being drawn off by the kidneys, before it is perfectly assimilated and applied to the purpose of nutrition (162)."

Before Matthew Dobson presented his results on a saccharine material in the urine of diabetic patients in 1776, he consulted with William Cullen, MD (1710-1790) who was a Scottish physician and chemist at the Edinburgh Medical School. Professor Cullen was one of the most famous medical scholars of his day who was the first to separate out diabetes mellitus and diabetes insipidus (164, 165). Thousands of patients consulted with Dr. Cullen in Edinburgh including the famous economist, Adam Smith (1723-1790) (167). Cullen noted a type of diabetes with urine having "the smell, color, and flavor of honey" versus diabetes with "limpid but not sweet urine" (167). Cullen advised Dobson: "You have done something in putting it beyond all doubt by your experiments... I have only to add that I wish you would examine both by taste and evaporation what might be called the Urina Potus or that copius limpid urine which runs in some people after their drinking largely of water or watery liquors" (164, 167).

Shortly after Matthew Dobson's work, Thomas Cawley noted that patients with pancreatic trauma developed diabetes and thus proposed a cause and effect in 1788; an example of injury to the pancreas was from stones as seen during an autopsy of a person with diabetes (10, 168). This observation ("near-miss") was neither appreciated nor understood until late into the next century!

Matthew Baillie (1761-1823)

Matthew Baillie (1761-1823) was a well-known Scottish physician and pathologist who came from a well-educated family and is noted by medical history for identifying situs inversus and transposition of the great arteries (169-172). The trio of Matthew Baille and is two famous uncles (William and John Hunger) have been called the founders of Great Britian's medicine.

Matthew Baille wrote the first classified book on pathology as its own topic and, as a pathologist, wrote:"...upon examination of the kidneys...it seemed probable that diabetes depends, in a considerable degree, upon a deranged action of the kidneys, by which the blood there is disposed to new combinations" the effect of which is the production of 'a saccharine matter'.... the chyle may be so imperfectly formed, as to make the blood be more readily changed into a saccharine matter, by the action of the kidneys" (172).

John Rollo (died 1809)

John Rollo was a Scottish military surgeon who became a consultant to patients with diabetes. In 1789 He used the term "mellitus" (Greek for honey: μέλι [meli]) to differentiate it from polyuria with no sugar and no taste ("insipidus") and felt that diabetes mellitus was a stomach disorder that developed from "vegetable substances containing saccharine matter" and this was promptly removed as a foreign body by the kidneys (10, 149, 173, 174). He utilized a urine glucose test developed by Matthew Dobson.

John Rollo wrote about increased sugar in the blood, an acetone odor on the breath of some diabetic patients and associated cataracts with diabetes (107). He recommended a meat diet (protein-rich, low carbohydrate) for management of diabetes mellitus that was used into the early 20th century (173, 174). He described his diet as high in "animal food" that was fat with meat ("plain blood puddings" with "rancid meat") as well as low in "vegetable matter (grains and breads)" (173, 174). Other therapeutic regimens included antimony, digitalis, and opium (107).

Table 7. 19th century giants in the history of diabetes

John Elliotson (1791-1868)
Michel Eugène Chevreuil (1786-1889)
John Elliotson (1791-1868)
Hermann von Fehling (1812-1885)
Claude Bernard (1813-1878)
William Prout (1785-1850)
Richard Bright (1789-1858)
Apollinaire Bouchardat (1806-1886)
Étienne Lancereaux (1829-1910)
Friedrich Theodor von Frerichs (1819-1885)
Adolf Kussmaul (1822-1902 AD)
Henry Noyes (1832-1900)
Edward Nettelship (1845-1913)
Bernard Naunyn (1840-1914)
Paul Langerhans (1847-1888)
Edouard Laguesse (1861-1927 AD)
Oscar Minkowski (1858-1931)
Joseph Freiherr von Mering (1849-1908)

PROGRESS IN THE 19TH CENTURY

A number of individuals contributed to the explosion of knowledge about diabetes in the 19th century (see Table 7). This includes Michel Eugène Chevreuil (1786-1889)—a famous and long-living French chemist with much fame for his work with fatty acids, creatine, and other scientific work (175-177). In 1815 he published his work that identified the sweet substance of Matthew Dobson's studies as being the same as grape sugar (i.e., glucose) (10, 149, 176). In 1849 German chemist Hermann von Fehling (1812-1885) developed a quantitative test (Fehling's solution) for glycosuria and the 19th century continued with an explosion of research on diabetes (10, 175, 176).

John Elliotson (1791-1868)

John Elliotson was a Scottish professor of medicine who was one of the early physicians to use a stethoscope. In his observation of patients with diabetes mellitus, which he concluded was a renal disorder, he noted possible etiologic factors that included "grief, chills, and excessive use of venery (149, 178)." He was an advocate for the use of phrenology and mesmerism in the treatment of human disease (179-181).

Claude Bernard (1813-1878)

A scientist whose works were translated into many languages and who is acclaimed in his native country and beyond is Claude Bernard, the most distinguished French physiologist of the 19th century (and beyond!) (98, 182). Though born to a poor family in the Beaujolais region of France and starting out to write theatre plays (la Rose du Rhône and Arthur de Bretagne), he rose to become chair of experimental physiology at the College de France (succeeding his mentor, François Magendie [1783-1855]) (46). Though honored by the Emperor Napoleon, Bernard was abandoned by his family over his experiments involving vivisection (46).

He accomplished many experiments in physiology that set the stage for sound scientific methodology and is acclaimed as the father of modern physiology and called by the eminent French microbiologist and chemist Louis Pasteur (1822-1895) as "physiology itself" (10, 98, 183). Bernard was willing to change his views based on science as illustrated by his initial idea that diabetes was a "nervous affection of the lungs" and later linking this disorder to the liver (46). He emphasized blind experiments to ensure scientific objectivity and he performed now classic experiments on the pancreas' function (i.e., discovered the lipolytic function of the exocrine pancreas) as well as the glycogenic function of the liver (with improvement in knowledge of diabetes mellitus) (98, 149, 155, 182-190).

Claude Bernard was the first to describe homeostasis or constancy of the internal environment (le milieu intèrieur) and the vasomotor system. This allowed future researchers to apply these principles to renal physiology. For example, research in the first half of the 20th century lead to the definition of electrolyte content of le milieu intérieur—the extracellular, intracellular, and interstitial fluid compartments (98, 191-193).

Claude Bernard identified his “starch-like” material (glycogen) that was a glucose precursor and alerted the medical community to the important role of the liver in its production and in diabetes (164). It was a major discovery that the sugar found in the diabetic patient’s urine was the stored in the liver and Bernard concluded that glycogenolysis led to diabetes; he concluded that sympathetic influence was important in this process as he was the discover of vasomotor innervation (46, 107, 149). In his work on dogs he was able to decrease their pancreatic masses but since they did not develop diabetes, he did not associate diabetes with a pancreatic disorder (194). However, his technique to ligate pancreatic ducts was utilized later by researchers to search for the cause of diabetes (10).

Claude Bernard wrote about the development of temporary glycosuria in animals after their fourth ventricle were punctured in a procedure he called “piqûre diabétique;” this transient state set the stage for the influence of the central nervous system and emotion on diabetes that was later identified (46, 155).

> The living organism does not really exist in the milieu exterieur (the atmosphere if it breathes, salt or fresh water if that is its element) but in the liquid milieu interieur formed by circulating organic liquid, which surrounds and bathes all tissue elements,...the stability of the milieu interieur is the primary condition for freedom and independence of existence; the mechanism which allows this is that which ensures in the milieu interieur the maintenance of all conditions necessary to the life of the elements.”
> Claude Bernard (190)

William Prout (1785-1850)

William Prout (1785-1850) was an acclaimed English physician (endocrinologist) and chemist known for the Prout’s hypothesis regarding the internal arrangement of the atom and identified hydrochloric acid as the acid of gastric secretion (195). He concluded that diabetes was a gastric disorder (196). He is known in the medical field for being the first person to identify diabetic coma (10,195-199). He hypothesized that etiologic factors in diabetes included “drinking of cold fluids when heated,” as well as “mental anxiety and distress” (195-202).

Richard Bright (1789-1858)

The 19th and 20th century brought forth brilliant scholars, who, standing on the shoulders of previous giants, advanced the field of clinical nephrology to its current level. Perhaps the beginning of modern nephrology can be traced to the Richard Bright (1789-1858) who has been called the "greatest physician of his day and one of five or six great physicians of all time" (98, 202). He was one of the famous triumvirate of London's Guy's Hospital in the Victorian era—along with Thomas Addison (1793-1860) and Thomas Hodgkin (1798-1866). Each of these three medical giants had diseases named after them.

This father of modern renal diseases noted that the finding of albuminuria with edema meant the patient had renal disease. The first clinical mention of proteinuria was in 1697 but it was Richard Bright who, standing on the shoulders of giants, moved this observation further in 1827(203,204). He established the first medical research unit at his hospital and provided a series of insightful descriptions of acute nephritis, nephrotic syndrome, uremia, small and enlarged kidneys, and a link between renal disease and enlarged ventricles of the heart (98, 205-210).

Acute and chronic nephritis was called Bright's disease long after his death that may have been caused by the very disease he described so well. Richard Bright's studies were often post-mortem on patients with advanced renal disease and his written observations are preserved in the Gordon Museum at London's Guy's Hospital (209). Analysis by late 20th century nephrologists revealed two had mesangiocapillary (membranoproliferative) glomerulonephritis; one had a five-year clinical history and died from chronic renal failure with uremia while the other died after 3 to 4 months with severe nephrotic syndrome (209). In his post-mortem observations of patients he concluded that diabetes was not due to renal disease but that the kidneys were affected by this condition—a concept affirmed in the 20th century (202).

Apollinaire Bouchardat (1806-1886)

Apollinaire Bouchardartis was a renowned French physician, biochemist, pharmacist, and hygienist. As a food crisis unfolded and many persons were starving during the Franco-Prussian war of 1870-1871, he noted that starvation reduced the glycosuria and other features of diabetes in patients with diabetes mellitus (107). His book, De la Glycosurie ou diabète sucré, son traitement hygénigue, is the first text on diabetes and was published in 1883; his advice to his diabetic patients was "mangez le moins possible" ("eat as little as possible") (211).

Bouchardartis is considered the founder of modern diabetology for his work on diet control of diabetes (with regular fasting and the Bouchardat's treatment with a low-carbohydrate meals), identifying the need for patient education as well as patient self-monitoring, development of a test for glycosuria used by the patient, stressing the importance of exercise, and correctly concluding that the etiology of diabetes was found in the pancreas (211-216).

Étienne Lancereaux (1829-1910)

Étienne Lancereaux (1829-1910) was a remarkable French physician who identified that diabetes was a condition of the pancreas and he used the term pancreatic diabetes (diabète pancréatique) after comparing the histology of pancreatic islet cells in those with and without diabetes (194, 217-219). He divided diabetes into two types: diabetes maigre (lean diabetes) and diabetes gras (fat diabetes) (217-219). The eponym Lancereaux's diabetes refers to diabetes mellitus with severe cachexia or emanciation. Not only was his pancreatic association of diabetes mellitus proven correct by later researchers (as considered later), but one of his students, Nicolae Paulescu (1869-1931) has been credited as one of the researchers who discovered insulin (220, 221).

Friedrich Theodor von Frerichs (1819-1885)

A large number of researchers and physicians attempted to further the knowledge of diabetes. A classic example of this movement was Friedrich Theodor von Frerichs (1819-1885); he was a German pathologist who developed a clinic for experimental medicine and wrote a treatise on diabetes mellitus (Über den Diabetes) in 1884 (202). In this work he noted that 20% of persons with diabetes had severe pathological pancreatic abnormalities (202). He had a number of students and assistants who made contributions to diabetes including Bernhard Naunyn (1840-1914, Paul Langerhans (1847-1888), and Paul Ehrlich (1854-1915). He provided a classic work on Bright's disease and provided information in hepatology, neurology (multiple sclerosis), and other fields (222-226). Slowly, but surely, diabetes was revealing its secrets and perplexities as the persistence of human curiosity and inquiry continued from century to century and from one medical giant to another.

Adolf Kussmaul (1822-1902)

Adolf Kussmaul was a German physician and teacher who provided a number of contributions to clinical medicine in his illustrious career that included neurology (i.e., progressive bulbar paralysis), endocrinology, cardiology (pulsus paradoxus), psychiatry, gastroenterology (developed gastric lavage; experimented with esophagoscopy as well as gastroscopy), and rheumatology (i.e., polyarteritis nodosa) (227-231). He is internationally known in diabetes for his classic description of typical air hunger (acidotic breathing) of diabetic ketoacidosis (232, 233). The puzzle of diabetes was being methodically assembled in this century. For example, Wilhelm Petters had identified in 1857 that acetone was found in the urine of those with diabetes (10). Adolf Kussmaul theorized that acetonemia caused the ketoacidotic coma in diabetes (10).

> Since I have seen three diabetics in the course of a year die, with remarkably similar symptoms in which there was a peculiar comatose condition preceded and accompanied by dyspnoea, I believe that it is not merely chance, but am of the opinion that it has to do with a form of death in diabetes which is rarely observed and bears the closest relationship to the disturbances in the metabolism in diabetes. (Adolf Kussmaul) (232)

Henry Noyes (1832-1900)

Henry Noyes was an American ophthalmologist who wrote two classic texts on eye diseases: A treatice on diseases of the eye (New York, 1881) and A textbook of diseases of the eye (New York, 1890, 2nd Edition: 1894). He invented a number of eye instruments still used today----such as the Noyes micro scissors, the Noyes iris scissors, and the Noyes fixation forcepts. Using the newly developed opthalmoscope, Henry Noyes wrote a paper in 1869 that noted patients with glycosuria develop retinitis and it was an early identification of diabetic retinopathy (10, 202, 234, 235). Finally, the Americans were chasing after the perplexities of diabetes!

A renowned British ophthalmologist, Edward Nettelship (1845-1913) confirmed this link with a seminar paper in 1872 showing histopathological evidence of "cystoid degeneration of the macula" in persons with diabetes; in 1877 he published a treatise on retinal pathology in these patients (235-239). Slowly but surely the pathology and complications of diabetes mellitus were being unravealed in the 19th century. Only some of these investigators are discussed in this book's edition, but addition heroes in this endeavor will be covered in future editions.

> The esteem and regard which Nettleship was universally held by his pupils and colleagues found definite expression at the date of his retirement from practice. The Fund then collected was, in accordance with his own desire, devoted to the establishment of a metal 'for the encouragement of scientific ophthalmic work.' This Prize is in the custody of the Opthalmological Society and is awarded triennially. In 1909, to the great satisfaction of all, it was awarded to Nettleship himself, in recognition of his researches upon the heredity of diseases of the eye. (Lancet, Nov 8, 1913) (238)

Bernard Naunyn (1840-1914)

Bernard Naunyn was a German pathologist who was born as well as trained in Berlin and, as noted, was a junior official to the imminent German pathologist, Friedrich Theodor von Frerichs (1819-1885) (222-226). He developed a clinic for persons with diabetes and wrote a book on this disorder in 1898 (240). Naunyn used the term "acidosis" in persons with diabetes mellitus and recommended the use of bicarbonate to manage this issue (10, 202, 240). He was part of the German Medical School of Strasbourg and worked with such luminaries as Oscar Minkowski and Joseph Freiherr von Mering to induce diabetes in dogs via pancreatectomy (155, 241). He also contributed to the link of psychological factors and diabetes by identifying a case of diabetes mellitus developing under the catastrophic circumstances of a city bombing (157). His work on drug metabolism, pharmacology, and cholelithiasis was also acclaimed (242).

Paul Langerhans (1847-1888)

Paul Langerhans was a German pathologist who studied under the famous father of pathology and social medicine, Rudolf Virchow (1821-1902) (243-251). As a medical student Paul Langerhans provided novel descriptions of tiny clusters of cells ("zellhaufen") from the pancreas not emptied by ducts of the pancreas (247). This finding was presented in his doctoral dissertation at the University of Berlin in 1869 that identified 9 types of cells in the pancreas based on his studies of the rabbit (249-251). He noted one set of pancreatic cells involved with normal pancreatic secretion and another set with unknown function (s). In our book "Chronic illness and disability: The pediatric pancreas," we present results of another doctoral dissertation on diabetes mellitus.

> Description of what was later called Islets of Langerhans by PaulLangerhans: "…kleine Zellen von meist ganz homogenem Inhalt und polygonaler mit rundern Kern ohne Kernkörpechen meist zu zweien oder zu kleinen Gruppen beisammen liegende." ("….small cells of almost perfect homogeneous content and of a polygonal form, with round nuclei without nucleoli, mostly lying together in pairs or small groups. (250)

Langerhans did not know the significance of these clusters though he speculated they may be lymph node or nerve tissue. He died in 1888 age at age 41 years before knowing their connection to insulin production and that they would be later be called islets of Langerhans by Edouard Laguesse (see below) and others. Paul Langerhans is a classic example of posthumous fame and honor. The inscription over his gravestone reads in Greek that is translated into English as: "Nor did my heart wish any longer to be alive and see the light of the sun." (248)

Edouard Laguesse (1861-1927)

Edouard Laguesse (Gustave François Antoine dit Édouard Laguesse) was a French physician, anatomist and histologist who identified the term, "endocrine," for the glands of internal secretion (252). In 1893 he theorized in that the pancreatic islands that were described by Paul Langerhans in 1869 that he called "les ilots de Langerhans" may be the basis or determinant of blood glucose control and were the endocrine glands or tissue of the pancreas (253-257).

CLOSE OF THE 19TH CENTURY: PSYCHOLOGICAL FACTORS

As the 19th century rushed to a close, the result of furious scientific experiments began to come to fruition. After thousands of years of confusion about the etiology, symptoms, and treatment for persons with diabetes mellitus, science was merging into a clearer understanding of this disorder. It was not a gastric nor renal disorder, but one of the pancreas. Psychological factors also play a role, as first revealed by Thomas Willis and Claude Bernard (157). William H Dickinson wrote in 1875 that diabetes was a disease of the nervous system that involved secretion of saccharine in the urine (202,258). Though departing from the growing sense in the later 19th century that diabetes was a pancreatic condition, it continued the notion that the nervous system and perhaps psychological factors were involved in this complex disorder (157).

Oscar Minkowski (1858-1931) and Joseph Freiherr von Mering (1849-1908)

Oscar Minkowski (1858-1931) was born in Alexoten (now in Lithuania) and his family moved to Königsberg (Prussia) 14 years after his birth. He studied medicine at the University of Königsberg and his interest in research as well as his surgical prowess would serve the cause of diabetes knowledge well (241). Joseph von Mering (Joseph Frieprich Freiherr von Mering; 1849-1908) was born in Cologne, Germany who became a physician and was involved in the discovery of the class of sedative drugs called barbiturates. His interest in the pancreas and his teaming up with Minkowski lead to a seminar progress in the field of diabetes.

Von Mering was visiting the library at the University of Strasbourgh and met Minkowski. Von Mering had been publishing on temporary glycosuria due to phloridzin which is a flavonoid found in apples, leaves, bark, and other naturally occurring tissues (46, 241). Von Mering had been looking at lipid digestion using an oil substance called Lipanin that contained free fatty acids

(46, 241). Their meeting with resultant communication led to their famous work in which Oscar Minkowski and Joseph Mereing were able to perform a pancreatectomy on a dog in 1889 and the dog lived but then developed fatal diabetes (46, 83, 106, 107, 154, 155, 259-264).

This was discovered after Minkowski looked for and found glycosuria in the urine left on the floor, because it had not been cleaned up after the dog developed polyuria (46, 149, 265). Since they were not sure if this was caused by this dog having been on phloridzin, these researchers performed pancreatectomy in three more dogs who did not have presurgical glycosuria, but who developed post-surgical glycosuria (46). Unlike the earlier experiments by Johann Conrad Brunner (1653-1727) as noted earlier, the Minkowski-Von Mering experiments on the canine pancreas stimulated others to seek to find the pancreatic substance linked with glucose metabolism (155, 157, 266). Minkowski and others also noted that when pancreatic tissue was added subcutaneously, glucose metabolism improved even if the pancreas was removed until the tissue was removed or became non-functional (46). Treatment of persons with diabetes mellitus was based on diet as championed by Bouchardat and others in the 19th century such as Ludwig Traube (1816-1876) advocating reduced carbohydrate intake (107, 266, 267).

> A dead thing can go with the stream, but only a living thing can go against it. Gilbert K Chesterton. (1874-1936)

REFULGANT DIABETES RESEARCH IN THE 20TH CENTURY

Standing on the shoulders of giants, medicine marches forward. Table 8 lists giants of the 20th century who marched medicine toward more definitive understanding of this disease that had perplexed homo sapiens for millennia. As noted earlier, the French physician and anatomist, Edouard Laguesse (1861-1927), in 1893 named the clusters of cells identified by Paul Langerhans in 1869 the "les ilots de Langerhans" and theorizied that they were involved in blood glucose control (248, 252-256). The Americans entered the study of diabetes with the work of the great 20th century pathologist, Eugene Lindsay Opie (1873-1971) (267-277). He was born in Virginia and grew up in Marland where he graduated from medical school at Johns Hopkins in Baltimore, Maryland.

Table 8. 20th century giants in the history of diabetes (Partial list)

Eugene Lindsay Opie (1873-1971)
Georg Ludwig Zuelzer (1870-1949)
Jean de Mayer (1878-1934)
Edward Albert Sharpey-Schafer (1850-1935)
Russell Lafayette Cecil MD (1881-1965)
Walter Bradford Cannon (1871-1945)
Sir Archibald E. Garrod (1857-1936)
Frederick Madison Allen (1878-1964)
Elliott Proctor Joslin (1869-1962)
Israel Kleiner (1885-1966)
Nicolae Constantine Paulescu (1869-1931)
Moses Barron (1884-1974)
Sir Frederick Grant Banting (1891-1941)
John James Rickard (JJR) Macleod (1876-1935),
Charles Herbert Best (1899-1978)
James Bertram Collip (1892-1965)
John Jacob Abel (1857-1938)
Sir Harold Himsworth (1905-1993),
Frederick Sanger (1918-2013
Hans Christian Hagedorn (1888-1971)
Donald Frederick Steiner (1930-2014)
Many others in the later part of the 20th century

Similar to the story of Paul Langerhans, Opie was a remarkable medical student and studied these clusters of cells. He know from previous scientists (i.e., von Mering, Merkowski, and Russian physician Leonid W. Ssobolew [1876-1919] and others) that complete blockage of pancreatic secreting ducts by pancreatic duct ligatiion did not lead to diabetes (271). It was also known that some type of "internal secretions" of the pancreas was involved in glucose metabolism.

In the very early 20th century Opie linked damage to the islets of Langerhans to diabetes and distinguished two forms of chronic insterstitial nephritis with islets that were damaged (272, 273). Eugene Opie went on to link damage to the islets of Langerhans to diabetes in 1901. He was able to distinguish two forms of chronic interstitial nephritis with damage islets. He wrote the first edition of "Diseases of the pancreas" in 1903. He noted that "Diabetes mellitus… is caused by destruction of the islands of Langerhans and occurs only when these bodies are in part or wholly destroyed" (274). His legacy in the field of diabetes lives on into the 21st century (149, 274-277).

> Modern scientific medicine, with its deep insight into the nature of disease, is capable of conferring immense benefit upon mankind. [Indeed] medicine offers one of the greatest opportunities to serve mankind. (Eugene Lindsay Opie (1873-1971) (268)

Early 20th century progress: 1900-1905

In addition to the work of Eugene Lindsay Opie (1873-1971), the first five years of the 20th century also provided research by the Russian physician, Leonid W Ssobolew (1876-1919), who ligated animal pancreatic ducts (i.e., rabbits, cats, and dogs) and noted this led to degeneration of enzyme-secreting acini cells; the islet cells were viable for weeks and diabetes did not result (278, 279). Other researchers were involved in such experiments, such as Schulze, in 1900 who independently reached the same result (278, 279).

Other progress was seen in 1902 when English physiologists Sir William Maddock Bayliss (1860-1924) and Ernest Henry Starling (1866-1927) revealed the concept of gastrointestinal peristalsis and the presence of a peptide bioactive substance called secretin in the gastrointestinal tract since it was secreted in the intestinal tract and regulated secretions of the pancreas and other organs; they introduced the term "hormone" for the first time in 1905 (280-284). They became well-known in the science community of the 20th and now 21st century for these and other achievements in physiology research. The role of secretin continued to be investigated to the present including potential role in managing obesity (283, 284).

Early 20th century progress: 1906-1910

Between 1906 and 1908 Georg Ludwig Zuelzer (1870-1949) was involved in early research on pancreatic extracts and diabetes. This physician in Berlin, Germany performed pancreatectomy on dogs and then injected the animals with pancreatic extracts which reduced glucose in their urines (10, 155, 202, 285-288). He developed a US patent on his alcoholic extract (called Acomatol), but intolerable side effects resulted from the use of the pancreatic digestive enzymes. The side effects included a convulsive reaction perhaps due to hypoglycemia (10). Though his extract did have a hypoglycemic effect, he did not continue with this research perhaps, as noted by some authorities, Zuelzer was not encouraged to pursue it partially due to the emergence of World War I.

However, Georg Ludwig Zuelzer was the first person in thousands of years to have partial success with a pancreatic extact (155). The secrets of the pancreas were slowly being understood. Scientists Michael Lane and RR Bensley identified the pancreatic ilets A and B cells in 1907 and 1911 respectively using improved histological methods (290, 291). Eventually it is found that the A (α) cells produce glucagon and the B (ß) cells produce insulin (292-294).

In 1909 Beglian physician Jean de Mayer (1878-1934) uses the term insulin (Latin for insulina or island) for the material in the ilets of Langerhans that many have concluded is in the pancreas and in agreement with concepts of previously mentioned, French anatomist/physician, Edouard Laguesse (1861-1927 AD), controls glucose metabolism.

Another scientiest, Scottish endocrinologist and physiologist Sir (knighted in 1913) Edward Albert Sharpey-Schafer (1850-1935) also independently proposes the name insulin for this pancreatic substance calling it "pro-insuline" in 1910 and theorized that diabetes is caused by a deficiency of this material that he called an antidiabetic chemical (295, 296). He has been called an important link in the development of endocrinology as a specialty of medicine. He is also known for contributions to the methodology of artificial respiration (297, 298).

Early 20th century progress: 1911-1920

One of the great American physicians and internists of the 20th century was Russell Lafayette Cecil, MD (1881-1965) (299-303). Early in his career he joined with other researchers and clinicians in 1911 who were linking damage of the islets of Langerhans to diabetes mellitus (304). He became well-known for his work on pneumonia, established concepts of controlled trials (clinical trials), and then starting in 1927 he edited what became one of the best known American textbooks of internal medicine (Cecils's textbook of medicine) that is now in its 25th edition despite his death in 1965 (303-311).

Table 9. Giants in the field of behavioral factors in diabetes mellitus (partial list)

Thomas Willis (1632-1675)
Claude Bernard (1813-1878)
Bernard Naunyn (1840-1914)
Walter Bradford Cannon (1871-1945)
Sir Archibald E. Garrod (1857-1936)

In 1911 Ernest L Scott at the University of Chicago reported that glycosuria in pancreatectomized dogs was "slightly" lowered after providing intravenous aqueous pancreatic extracts. In the same unfortunate milieu as experienced by Georg Ludwig Zuelzer (1870-1949) a few years ea rlier, Scott's experiments of 1911 and 1912 were dismissed as being unimportant and the discovery of insulin had to wait another ten years (287, 288). His mentors suggested this mild reduction in urine glucose was "doubtless explained by renal or other nonspecific changes (287, 288)." Ernest L Scott was in the right direction but stopped short of the goal of finding insulin and his work became another near-miss in the search for effective management of diabetes mellitus (312).

EMOTIONAL GLYCOSURIA

As researchers were unfathoming the mysteries of diabetes in the second decade of the 20th century, the influence of emotion and psychological factors on diabetes was also being explored (see Table 9). As noted earlier in this treatise, a link of emotion and diabetes was identified by the 17th century British physician/anatomist, Thomas Willis (1632-1675) (149, 157). This association was also explored by the great French physiologist of the 19th century, Claude Bernard (1813-1878) (46, 157). Also, as noted earlier the German pathologist Bernard Naunyn (1840-1914) wrote about diabetes developing during the stressful milieu of war with bombing of a city in 1870 (157).

The German term, "Fesselungs diabetes" arose from the experiments of German researchers Boehm and Hoffmann who published their work in 1878 about the appearance of glycosuria within 30 minutes in cats who were fastened to a board and were tracheotomized without anesthesia (313). A researcher who would receive the Nobel Prize in 1923 noted in 1907 that the amount of sugar in the blood was controlled by afferent and efferent nerve fibers (314).

In 1911 this link was further developed by the work of the great American physiologist, Walter Bradford Cannon (1871-1945), who became of considerable fame from various experiments and ideas including his identification of the fight or flight response and furthered the concept of Claude Bernard's concepts of homeostatis in human beings (315-319). Cannon agreed and confirmed the Fesselungs glycosuria found by Boehm and Hoffmann but he did not feel that the glycosuria was due to pain or being bound; instead, he felt that this physiologic effect was due to metabolic effects induced by the fight or flight response and that this stress led to sympathetic nervous system stimulation with an increase in epinephrine (157, 320, 321).

Cannon advanced the concept of "emotional" glycosuria and connected it to the sympathetic nervous system. Some researches noted in 1911 that emotional glycosuria can be due to stress-induced hypervention that leads to acapnia (322). The English physician, Sir Archibald E Garrod (1857-1936), father of the field of inborn errors of metabolism (323, 324), concluded in 1912 that "psychic strain or stress" was a contributing factor in emotional glycosuria (157, 325). In 1914 researchers O Folin, W. Denis, and WG Smillie published their observations in which medical and college students developed transient glycosuria under the stress of examinations (326).

Frederick Madison Allen (1879-1964)

Frederick Madison Allen was an American physician best remembered for his promotion of a carbohydrate-restricted/high fat diet in the second decade of the 20th century for management of diabetes mellitus (327-331). It proved to be a desperate measure that improved the glycosuria of some but this so-called "starvation diet" (70% fat, 8% carbohydrate) led to the deaths of others (331-333).

Elliott Proctor Joslin (1869-1962)

Elliott P Joslin became the leading specialist in diabetes mellitus in the 20th century and was the first physician to fully specialize in one disease as diabetes (334,335). His interest in metabolism began in the 19th century and, before insulin was available, agreed with Frederick Madison Allen (1889-

1964) that a restricted diet was helpful to patients with diabetes mellitus (332, 336). In the second decade of the 20th century he began to write about management of diabetes mellitus and in 1916 wrote a monograph "The treatment of diabetes mellitus" followed by his 1918 "Diabetic manual"—for the doctor and patient (337, 338). These works went into many editions as he established the Joslin Diabetes Center in Boston as a major institute for the study and treatment of diabetes mellitus (338). He was an advocate for patient education and tight glucose control—an approach noted later in the 20th century to be the correct one for maximal health and longevity of the person with diabetes mellitus.

> A patient needs a doctor, not a committee....Doctors treated individuals, not statistical averages...If you don't examine the trees, you may get lost in the woods. The proper study of mankind is man. (John P Peters, MD, 1887-1955) (98)

Israel Kleiner (1885-1966)

Between 1915 and 1919 researcher Israel Kleiner (1885-1966) was injecting pancreatic extracts into depancreatized animals and measuring the reduction in the blood sugar at the Rockefeller Institute in New York City (287, 288, 339-342). His work confirmed that a substance in the pancreas was involved in glucose control but his injections caused potential severe adverse effects and he was not able to find this purified substance.

> The result is regarded as further evidence for the internal secreation theory of experimental diabetes. Israel Kleiner (339)

Nicolae Constantine Paulescu (1869-1931)

Nicholas Paulesco was a professor of physiology in the Romanian School of Medicine (Bucharest, Romania) who performed research on dogs in the middle of the second decade of the 20th century seeking to identify the pancreatic extract substance that was involved in glucose metabolism (287, 288, 342-346). In August of 1921 he reported his results on a pancreatic substance he called "pancrein" and noted it lowered blood sugar in dogs (347).

For a variety reasons involving controversy and the interruption of World War I, Nicolae Paulescu was not given official recognition for his findings and this was given to Frederick Banting and colleaues in Toronto, Canada as discussed in the next section. Some scholars, including those in his home country, feel that this professor did not receive the recognition he should have and the readers of this book can research this issue and make up their own minds in this regard (270, 287, 342, 344-352).

> There is a tide in the affairs of men
> Which taken at the flood, leads on to fortune;
> Omitted, all the voyage of their life
> Is bound in shallows and in miseries. —
> Shakespeare, Julius Caesar, act iv, scene 3

Sir Frederick Grant Banting (1891-1941)

Frederick Grant Banting was a young Canadian orthopedic surgeon who had served heroically in World War I, where he was wounded and given credit by history as the discoverer of insulin though with some controversy as previously noted (353-357). The typically story that is "told" is that before giving a talk on diabetes in London (Ontario, Canada), he read an article by Moses Barron published in 1920 that had an important, seminal reflection that diabetes was not found in persons with pancreatic disease if the pancreatic islets were not involved (149, 356, 357). Moses Barron (1884-1974) was a physician and researcher born in Russia and grew up in Minnesota, USA. He also served in World War I and received the 1964 Banting Award from the American Diabetes Association (358,359).

In his classic 1920 article there was the discussion of a pancreas with fibrosis with intact islet cells but absent acinar cells and absent diabetes mellitus; the paper also provided citations of others' research with similar results from pancreatic duct ligation (267, 357, 358). Moses Barron discussed his work in article in Minnesota Medicine (1966; 49:689). This work relates to that of French physician and anatomist, Eugene Lindsay Opie (1873-1971) (271-278), Russian physician Leonid W Ssobolew [1876-1919] (271,278), and others as previous reviewed in this article.

The inspiration of reading this article led Sir Frederick Banting to talk to one of the great carbohydrate experts of his time, Professor John James Rickard (JJR) Macleod (1876-1935), an Aberdonian Scott who emigrated to

Canada; Banting asked for the use of a laboratory to carry out experiments he had in mind that included ligation of canine pancreatic ducts (287,350). Though described as skeptical JJR Macleod provided this young inexperienced researcher (Banting) with a laboratory, some dogs (Scottish border collies), and a laboratory assistant at the Toronto General Hospital. Banting went to work that night and two lab assistants were available and so a coin toss picked medical student Charles Herbert Best (1899-1978)—later elevating this American-Canadian to the glory as a co-discoverer of insulin and the other lab assistant to Shakespearean obscurity (288,357,360).

> There is a tide in the affairs of men
> Which taken at the flood, leads on to fortune;
> Omitted, all the voyage of their life
> Is bound in shallows and in miseries. —
> Shakespeare, Julius Caesar, act iv, scene 3

Much has been written about the details of the Banting-Best experiments (10, 107, 287, 288, 342). A classic description is by Banting himself, including that given on September 15, 1925 as his Nobel lecture given in Stockholm (288). The publications of Professor John JR Mccleod are also helpful in this regard (361-363) as well other publications by Banting and Best (364, 365). The key was finding an extract from the pancreas that would safely lower blood sugar in human beings. Initial extracts would produce unacceptable advere effects such as fever.

The breakthrough came when JJR Macleod, instead of giving up on the experiments and joining in a long line of "near-misses" in diabetes research, added a chemist to the Toronto group destined for medical glory--- James Bertram Collip (1892-1965)---a biochemist who could purify a crude alcohol pancreatic extract, keep it cool on ice, and added the seminal idea of using beef pancreatic extracts as well as effects of the extracts in rabbits to help meansure the glucose lowering potential to avoid an insulin overdose (164, 287, 364-366).

After working with pancreatectomized dogs the breakthrough patient was 14 year old Leonard Thompson (1908-1935) with type 1 diabetes mellitus who developed an allergic reaction to the original Banting-Best pancreatic extract given on January 11, 1922 but did well with the extract refined by biochemist James Collip and given 12 days later; this patient lived to age 27 years and died from pneumonia (149, 267, 342). Banting and Macloud received the 1923 Nobel Prize for their discovery of insulin and Banting provided public recognition for Charles Best (sharing the Nobel Prize with him) and Macloud did the same for James Collip (166, 362).

Macleod provided his thoughts on the action of this hypoglycemic compound in his 1925 Nobel Lecture and wondered about its mechanism---a question that would take many decades in the 20th century to answer (361). Clashes of personalities led to the Toronto team dissolving and others taking leadship in diabetes management advances in the 20th century—perhaps accentuated by post-tramatic stress issues with Banting as a WWI veteran (349). Frederick Banting died in 1941 in a plane crash. As noted, history has clouded the Toronto group with considerable controvery and the reader can decide what is valid and what is not (267, 287, 342, 344-352). Certainly their success followed the work of others in the past (202).

However, the mantel of glory is generally given to this Toronto group whose discovery that insulin is secreted in the beta cells of the pancreas went on to save millions and millions of lives in the 20th and now 21st century (107, 342). Frederick Banting was knighted in 1934. Certainly sharing in the glory of insulin discovery and purification is the pharmaceutical industry (i.e., Connaught Laboratories, Eli Lilly and Company, and Nordisk Insulin Laboratory) who made a safe insulin product available to the public within months of this discovery (149, 164, 166).

> Mine is the first step and therefore a small one, though worked out with much thought and hard labor. You, my readers or hearers of my lectures, if you think I have done as much as can fairly be expected of an initial start. . . will acknowledge what I have achieved and will pardon what I have left for others to accomplish. Aristotle.
> (385 BC-322 BCE)

POST-BANTING/BEST ERA

Sir Henry Hallett Dale (1875-1968) was an English pharmacologist who was involved in organizing scientific meetings in 1923 and 1925 to develop international standards for insulin and other biological agents; he established the National Institute for Medical Research to establish these critically important standards (368). Henry H Dale received a Nobel Prize in 1936 for his work on acetylcholine. John Jacob Abel (1857-1938) was a biochemist and pharmacologist with an MD degree who chaired the first department of pharmacology at the Univeristy of Michigan and then was chair of pharmacology at Johns Hopkins University (369, 370). He purified insulin and identified its crystalline structure in 1926 (164, 369). In 1936 Sir Harold Himsworth (1905-1993), a professor of medicine at London University, identified two types of diabetes mellitus—insulin-sensitive (type 1) and insulin-insensitive (insulin resistance, type 2) (371-374).

The term, insulin, came from the Latin word, "insula" for island (149). Further work on the insulin molecule occurred as the 20th century continued by double Nobel prize winner, British biochemist Frederick Sanger (1918-2013)---he identified the molecular structure of insulin in the 1940s and 1950s including the amino acid sequence of the protein insulin (164, 267, 375-377). Prior to that Protamine zinc insulin was introduced in the 1930s and neutral protamine Hagedorn (NPH) insulin in the late 1930s and early 1940s. Hans Christian Hagedorn (1888-1971) was a Danish physician who was influential in obtaining the legal rights for insulin from Banting and Best, developed NPH insulin, and helped form a company for insulin production now called Novo Nordisk (378-380).

Research in the 1940s and 1950s led to insulin syringes, urine testing methods (i.e., tablets, test strips), blood-glucose testing strips beginning in 1962, and oral sulfonylureas starting in 1958. Giants of medicine and research continued to come in the 20th century as noted with American physician and biochemist Donald Frederick Steiner (1930-2014) who discovered proinsulin at the University of Chicago in 1965 that allowed production of more pure insulin with less adverse effects (381).

Insulin pumps improved in the 1970s from earlier pumps by being portable and were complemented by new blood-glucose meters. The 1970s also saw the availability of U-100 insulin in 1973 and the first recombinant DNA insulin (1978). Research in the 1970s and 1980s ushered in the first biosynthetic human insulin that led in 1996 to FDA approval of the first recombinant DNA human insulin analog, lispro (Humalog). Simple-to-use insulin pens arrived in 1986 and self-monitoring of blood glucose was advancing from the 1980s into the 21st century.

The last decade of the 20th century and the early 21st century saw the fruition of years of research with new medications for type 2 diabetes including metformin, acarbose, repaglinide, and others (382, 383). Research continues to explore the mechanisms of the pancreas on glucose metabolism (384), the impact of diet on glucose control (385), management of gestational diabetes mellitus (386), genetic factors in diabetes (387), the potential association of diabetes mellitus with statins (388), control of hypertension in persons with diabetes (389), and the role of the gastrointestinal flora in diabetes management (390). Future issues of this book can detail 21st century advances that include different insulin delivery systems (i.e., inhalation, patch), improved insulins, genetic engineering to develop insulin-secreting cells, pancreatic transplantation, and others amazing advances (391-393).

> No human being is constituted to know the truth, the whole truth, and nothing but the truth; and even the best of men must be content with fragments, with partial glimpses, never the full fruition.
> (William Osler MD:1849-1919)

FINAL CHAPTER DENOUEMENT

> To suffer woes which Hope thinks infinite;
> To forgive wrongs darker than death or night;
> To defy Power, which seems omnipotent;
> To love, and bear; to hope till Hope creates
> From its own wreck the thing it contemplates;
> Neither to change, nor falter, nor repent;
> This, like thy glory, Titan, is to be
> Good, great and joyous, beautiful and free;
> This is alone Life, Joy, Empire, and Victory.
> Percy Bysshe Shelley's Prometheus Unbound, 1820

The current and future shortage of pediatric endocrinologists necessitates steady, rejuvenated information on diabetes and other endocrine disorders for primary care clinicians as they care for the child and adolescent with complex endocrine dilemmas and disorders (394-396). In view of this shortage and the rapidly increasing knowledge in pediatric diabetes as well understanding indications for referral to pediatric endocrinologists in the 21st century, au courant assiduous information aimed at primary care clinicians in these areas becomes increasingly important (397-400).

> Mine is the first step and therefore a small one, though worked out with much thought and hard labor. You, my readers or hearers of my lectures, if you think I have done as much as can fairly be expected of an initial start. . . will acknowledge what I have achieved and will pardon what I have left for others to accomplish.
> Aristotle (385 BC-322 BCE)

REFERENCES

[1] Early modern homo sapiens. URL: http://anthro.palomar.edu/homo2/mod_homo_4.htm.

[2] Magner LN. A history of the life sciences, 3rd ed. New York: Marcel Dekker, 2002.

[3] Kramer SN. The Sumerians. Chicago: The University of Chicago Press, 1963:225-6.

[4] Jastrow M. The liver in antiquity and the beginnings of anatomy. Tranasactions Coll Physicians 1907;XXIX:117.

[5] Roth MT. Law collections from Mesopotamia and Asia Minor. Atlanta, GA: Scholars Press, 1997.

[6] Geller MJ, Horstmanshoff HFJ, Stol M, Tilburg C, eds. West Meets East: Early Greeks and Babylonian diagnosis. Magic and rationality in ancient Near Eastern and Graeco-Roman Medicine. Boston, MA: Brill Publishers, 2004.

[7] Taylor JH, ed. Ancient Egyptian book of the dead: Journey through the afterlife. London: British Museum Press, 2010:54.

[8] Hallmann-Mikolajczak A. Ebers papyrus. The book of the medical knowledge of the 16th century BC Egyptians. Arch Hist Filoz Med 2004;67(1):5-14. [Polish].

[9] Stiefel M, Shaner A, Schaefer SD. The Edwin Smith papyrus: The birth of analytical thinking in medicine and otolaryngology. Laryngoscope 2006;116(2):182-8.

[10] Zajac J, Shrestha A, Patel P, Poretsky L. The main events in the history of diabetes mellitus. In: Poretsky L, ed. Principles of diabetes mellitus. New York: Springer Science, 2002:1-16.

[11] Loukas M, Lanteri A, Ferrauiola J, Tubbs RS, Maharaja G, Shoja MM, et al. Anatomy in ancient India: a focus on the Susruta Samhita. J Anat 2010;217(6):646-50.

[12] Frank LL. Diabetes mellitus in the texts of old Hindu medicine (Charaka, Susruta, Vagbhata). Am J Gastroenterol 1957;27(1):76-95.

[13] Sharma HS, Sharma HI, Sharma HA. Sushruta-samhitA: A critical review part-I: historical glimpse. Ayu 2012;33(2):167-73.

[14] Codellas PS. Alcmaeon of Croton: his life, work, and fragments. Proceed Royal Soc Med 1931;25(4):1041-6.

[15] Schiefsky MJ. Hippocrates: On ancient medicine. Leiden, Netherlands: Brill Publishers, 2005.

[16] Unguru S, Fried MN. Apollonius, Davidoff, Rorty, and Zeuthen: from A to Z, or, what else is there? Sudhoffs Arch 2007;91(1):1-19.

[17] André J. Remarks on the translation of Greek words into medical texts of the fifth century (Cassius Felix et Caelius Aurelianus). Rev Philol Litt Hist Anc 1963;37:47-67. [French].

[18] Coturri E. Surgery in Aurelianus Caelius [Vari XXXX]. Minerva Med 1959;50(35):Varia 898-914. [Italian].

[19] Saba MM, Ventura HO, Saleh M, Mehra MR. Ancient Egyptian medicine and the concept of heart failure. J Card Fail 2006;12(6):416-21.

[20] Van Praagh R, Van Praagh S. Aristotle's "triventricular" heart and the relevant history of the cardiovascular system. Chest 1983;84(4):462-8.

[21] Loukas M, Hanna M, AlsaieMason Stephen F. gh N, Shoja MM, Tubbs RS. Clinical anatomy as practiced by ancient Egyptians. Clin Anat 2011;24(4):409-15.
[22] Witters LA, Luciano M, Williams C, Yang J. Diabetes detectives. Dartmouth Med 2008;Winter:1-2.
[23] Wilson JC. Aulus Cornelius Celsus and some remarks concerning rare editions of old books and medical libraries. Bull Med Libr Assoc 1913;3(1):1-10.
[24] Androutsos G. Urology in the work De re medical of Aulus Cornelius Celsus (1st century AD). Prog Urol 2005;15(2):344-52. [French].
[25] Trancas B, Borja Santos N. Ethics, knowledge and psychiatry: in Aulus Cornelius Celsus' De Medicina. Acta Med Port 2007;20(5):431-7. [Portuguese].
[26] Finlayson J. Galen: [A bibliographical demonstration in the library of the faculty of physicians and surgeons of Glasgow, December 9th, 1891.]. Br Med J 1892;1(1628):573-5.
[27] Kempf EJ. From Hippocrates to Galen. Med Library Hist J 1904;2(4):282-307.
[28] Larkey SV. Galen: Greek, medievalist and modern: Part II. Cal West Med 1931;34(5):366-9.
[29] Hankinson RJ. Galen on Hippocratic physics. Stud Anc Med 2016;46:421-43.
[30] Kühn CG, ed. Claudii Galeni Opera Omnia. Leipzig: C Cnobloch, 1821.
[31] Bujalkova M. Rufus of Ephesus and his contribution to the development of anatomical nomenclature. Acta Med Hist Adriat 2011;9(1):89-100.
[32] Eknoyan G. Rufus of Ephesus and his "Diseases of the kidneys." Nephron 2002;91(3):383-90.
[33] Adams F, ed. Arataeus the Cappadocian: the extant works. London: Sydenham Society, 1856.
[34] Roselli A. Arataeus of Cappadocia's reading of the Hippocratic Corpus. Stud Anc Med 2005;31:413-32. [Italian].
[35] Laios K, Karamanou M. Saridaki Z, Androutsos G. Arataeus of Cappadocia and the first description of diabetes. Hormones (Athens) 2012;11(1):109-13.
[36] Garcia-Albea Ristol E. Arataeus of Cappadociaa (2nd century D) and the earliest neurological descriptions. Rev Neurol 2009;48(6):322-7. [Spanish].
[37] Tekiner H. Arataeus of Cappadocia and his treatises on diseases. Turk Neurosurg 2015;25(3):508-12.
[38] Reed JA. Arataeus the Cappadocian: History enlightens the present. Diabetes 1954;3:419-21.
[39] Greydanus DE, Hofmann AD. Psychological factors in diabetes mellitus: a review of the literature with emphasis in adolescence. Am J Dis Child 1979;133:1061-6.
[40] Cordell EF. Arateus of Cappadocia. Bull Johns Hopkins Hosp 1909;20:371-7.
[41] Pearce JMS. The neurology of Arateus: Radix pedis neuralgia. Eur Neurol 2013;106-112.
[42] Bongartz LG, Cramer J, Joles JA. Origins of the cardiorenal syndrome and the cardiorenal connection. Chronic Kidney Disease. URL: http://cdn..intechopen.com/pdfs-wm/32307/pdf.
[43] Kirchhof M, Popat N, Malowany J. A historical perspective of the diagnosis of diabetes. Univ West Ontario Med J 2008;78(1):1-4.

[44] Guthrie DW, Humpheys SS. Diabetes urine testing: an historical perspective. Diabetes Educ 1988;14(6):521-6.
[45] Laron Z. Childhood diabetes towards the 21st century. J Pediatr Endocrinol Metabol 1998;11(3):387-402.
[46] Karamanou M, Protogerou A, Tsoucalas G, Androutsos G, Poulakou-Rebelakou E. Milestones in the history of diabetes mellitus: The main contributors. World J Diabetes 2016;7(1):1-7.
[47] Bestetti RB, Baraldi C, Restini BA, Couto LB. Development of anatomophysiologic knowledge regarding the cardiovascular system: from Egyptians to Harvey. Arq Bras Cardiol 2014;103(6):538-45.
[48] Christopoulou-Aletra H, Papavramidou N. 'Diabetes' as describe by Byzantine writers from the fourth to the ninth century AD: the Graeco-roman influence. Diabetologia 2008;51(5):892-6.
[49] Baldwin B. The career of Oribasius. Acta Cl 1975;18:85-97.
[50] Riou YF. Un fragment d'un manuscript disparu d'Oribase, C.L.A. 116 (Vatican, Urb. lat. 293, ff. 95-96, VIIIe siècle). Scriptorium 1979;33:235-7.
[51] Lascaratos J, Poulakou-Rebelakou E. Oribasius (fourth Century) and early Byzantine perinatal nutrition. J Pediatr Gastroenterol Nutr 2003;36(2):186-9.
[52] Mikic Z. Famous physicians from the past—Oribasisus from Pergamum. Med Pregl 2013;66(3-4):189-92. [Serbian].
[53] Shirodkar JA, Sayyad MG, Nanal VM, Yajnik CS. Anguli parimana in Ayurveda and its association with adiposity and diabetes. J Ayurveda Integr Med 2014;5(3):177-84.
[54] Irmer D. Bearbeitungen von Schriften des iatrosophisten palladius unter den namen des Johannes, Stephanus, und Theophilus. Medizinhist J 1973;8(2-3):179-81. [German].
[55] Papathanassiou MK. Stephanus of Alexandria: pharmaceutical notions and cosmology in his alchemical work. Ambix 1990;37(3):121-33.
[56] Papathanassiou MK. Stephanus of Alexandria; on the structure and date of his alchemical work. Med Secoli 1996;8(2):247-66.
[57] Bouras-vallianatos P. Clinical experience in late antiquity: Alexander of Tralles and the therapy of epilepsy. Med Hist 2014;58(3):337-53.
[58] Puschmann T. Nachträge zu Alexander Trallianus. Fragmente aus philumenus und philagrius, nebst einer Bisher noch ungedruckten abhandlung über augenkrankheiten. Berlin: Verlag von S Calvary, 1886. [German].
[59] Delisle L, Le cabinet des manuscrits de la Bibliothèque nationale, 4 tomes, Paris, Imprimerie Nationale, 1868-1891 (réimpression 1978).
[60] Ongaro G. Le conoscenze elmintologiche de Alessandro di Tralle. Acta Med Hist Patav 1964-5;11:119-43. [Italian].
[61] Nutton V.The Latin Alexander Trallianus: the text and transmission of a Latin medical book (review). Bull Hist Med 2009;83(2):388-9.
[62] Papavramidou N, Christopoulou-Aletra H. Greco-Roman and Byzantine views on obesity. Obes Surg 2007;17(1):112-6.

[63] Mylonas AI, Poulakou-Rebelakou EF, Androutsos GI, Seggas I, Skouteris CA, Papadopoulou EC. Oral and cranio-maxillofacial surgery in Byzantium. Craniomaxillofac Surg 2014;42(2):159-68.
[64] Poulakou-Rebelakou E, Marketos SG. Kidney disease in Byzantine medical texts. Am J Nephrol 1999;19(2):172-6.
[65] Diamandopoulos A. Twelve centuries of nephrological writings in the Graeco-Roman world of the Eastern Mediterranean (from Hippocrates to Aetius Amidanus). Nephrol Dial Transplant 1999;14(Suppl 2):2-9.
[66] Scarborough J. Teaching surgery in late Byzantine Alexandria. Stud Anc Med 2010;35:235-60.
[67] 67 Sideras A. Aetius und Oribasius: Ihre gemeinsamen Exzerpte aus der Schrift des Rufus von Ephesos "Ueber die Nieren- und Blasenleiden" und ihr Abhängigkeitsverhältnis. Byzantinische Z 1974;67:110-30. [German].
[68] Conti Bizzarro F. Per l'edizione dei libri medicinali di Aezio Amideno. Koinonia 1978;2:169-97. [Italian].
[69] Durling RJ. Addenda lexicis, primary from Aëtius of Amida and Paul of Aegina. Glotta 1986;44(1-2):30-6.
[70] Lascaratos J, Tsirou M, Fronimopoulos J. Ophthalmology according to Aetius Amidenus. Doc Ophthalmol 1990;74(1-2):37-48.
[71] Karenberg A, Hort I. Medieval descriptions and doctrines of stroke: preliminary analysis of select sources. Part I: The struggle for terms and theories—late antiquity and early Middle Ages. J Hist Neurosci 1998;7(113 Pt 2):162-73.
[72] Gamillscheg E. Copyists of manuscripts for medicine. Med Secoli 1999;11(3):477-86. [German]
[73] Ramoutsaki IA, Dimitriou H, Kalmanti M. Management of childhood diseases in the Byzantine period: I—analgesia. Pediatr Int 2002;44(3):335-7.
[74] Bieganowski L. Ophthalmology in Byzantium between the 4th and the 7th century. Klin Oczna 2005;107(1-3):177-81. [Polish]
[75] Mylonas AI, Poulakou-Rebelakou EF, Androutsos GI, Seggas I, Skouteris CA, Papadopoulou EC. Oral and cranio-maxillofacial surgery in Byzantium. J Craniomaxillofac Surg 2014;42(2):159-68.
[76] Francis A. The medical works of Paulus Aegineta, the Greek physician: Translated into English with a copious commentary containing a comprehensive view of the knowledge possessed by the Greeks, Romans, and Arabians, on all subjects connected with medicine and surgery. First Edition. London: Welsh Treuttel Würtz, 1834. Book found in the collections of Oxford University. URL: https://archive.org/details/medicalworkspau00paulgoog.
[77] Pormann PE. The oriental tradition of Paul of Aegina's Pragmateia. Stud Anc Med 2004;29:1-337.
[78] Coturri E. Considerations on the surgical doctrinaire of Paul of Aegina. Minerva Med 1959;50:1665-8. [Italian].
[79] Gurunluoglu R, Gurunluoglu A. Paulus Aegineta, a seventh century encyclopedist and surgeon: his role in the history of plastic surgery. Plast Reconstruc Surg 2001;108(7):2072-9.
[80] Lascaratos J, Cohen M. Paul of Aegina. Plast Reconstr Surg 2002;110(5):1600-1.

[81] Papadakis M, de Bree E, Trompoukis C, Manios A. Paul of Aegina's surgical instruments: a complete surgical instrumentarium in the seventh century AD. Anz J Surg 2015 Mar 2. doi:10.1111/ans.13027.
[82] Peumery JJ. Histoire illustrée du diabète. De l'Antiquitéa nos jours. Paris: Roger Dacosta, 1987.
[83] Eknoyan G, Naby J. A history of diabetes mellitus or how a disease of the kidneys evolved into a kidney disease. Adv Chronic Kidney Dis 2005;12(2):223-9.
[84] Needham J, Lu G-D. Proto-endocrinology: Medieval preparations of urinary steroid and protein hormones. Science and Civilization in China, Volume 5: Chemistry and chemical technology, Part 5: Spagyrical discovery and invention. Physiological alchemy, Cambridge, UK: Cambridge University, 1983:301-37.
[85] Androutsos G. Theophilus Protospatharius: Byzantine forerunner of urology. Hist Sci Med 2007;41(1):41-8. [French].
[86] Gorgieva GS. Kidney disease in medieval Serbian manuscripts from the Chilandar monastery (Mount Athos, Greece). J Nephrol 2006;19(Suppl 10):S30-7.
[87] Iorio L, Lamagna M. Foam in urine: from Hippocrates to the medical school of Salerno. G Ital Nefrol 2014;31(2). pii: gin/31.2.14. [Italian]
[88] Theophilus: De urinis. Édition gréco-latine. Traduction par Thomas Guidot, 1703.
[89] Touwaide A. Sephanus of Athens. The encyclopedia of ancient history, 2012. doi: 1002/9781444338386.wbeah21306.
[90] Nutton V. Stepanus of Athens, Commentary on Hippocrates' Aphorisms, Section 1-2, Corpus Medicorum Graecorum XI 1,3,1. Med Hist 1986;30(2):228-9.
[91] Westerink Leendert G, ed. Stepanus of Athens, Commentary on Hippocrates' Aphorisms, Section III-IV, Corpus Medicorum Graecorum XI 1,3,2. Berlin: Akademie Verlag, 1992.
[92] Westerink Leendert G, ed. Stepanus of Athens, Commentary on Hippocrates' Aphorisms, Section V-VI, Corpus Medicorum Graecorum XI 1,3,3. Berlin: Akademie Verlag, 1995.
[93] Garofalo I. The Arabic translations of Alexandrian compendia of the works of Galen's Canon. The ad glauconem compendium. Med Secoli 1994;6(2):329-48. [Italian].
[94] Angeletti LR, Cavarra B. The Peri ouron treatise of Stephanus of Athens: Byzantine uroscopy of the 6th-7th centuries AD. Am J Nephrol 1997;17(3-4):228-32.
[95] Flaws B, L Kurchinski L, Casanas RJ. The treatment of diabetes mellitus with Chinese medicine: A textbook and clinical manual. Boulder, CO: Blue Poppy Press, 2002.
[96] Bowersock G. The vanishing paradigm of the Fall of Rome. Bull Amer Acad Arts Sciences 1996;49(8):29–43.
[97] Masic I, Dilic M, Solakovic E, Rustemepasic N, Ridjanovic Z. Why historians of medicine called Ibn al-Nafis the second Avicenna? Med Arh 2008;62(4):244-9.
[98] Greydanus DE, Raj VMS, Merrick J. From the Kition, Cyprus and Aristotelian kidney to the 21st century pediatric kidney: standing on the shoulders of giants. In: Greydanus DE, Raj VMS, Merrick J, eds. Chronic illness and disability: The pediatric kidney. New Yok: Nova Biomedical, 2016:3-26.
[99] Eknoyan G. Arabic medicine and nephrology. Am J Nephrol 1994;14:270-8.

[100] Changizi Astivani S, Shamsi M, Cyrus A, Bastani B, Tabatabayei SM. A critical review of the works of pioneer physicians on kidney diseases in ancient Iran: Avicenna, Rhazes, Al-akhawayni, and Jorjani. Iran J Kidney Dis 2011;5(5):300-8.
[101] Dunea G. History of nephrology: beginnings. Hektoen Internat: J Med Humanities. URL: http://www.hektoeninternational.org/index/php?option=com.
[102] Muntner Z. Persian medicine and its relation to Jewish and other medical science; commemorating the millennium of Avicenna. Harofe Haivri Heb Med J 1951;2:171-6.
[103] Chamsi-Pasha MAR, Chamsi-Pasha H. Avicenna' contribution to cardiology. Avicenna J Med 2014;4(1):9-12.
[104] Faridi P, Zarshenas MM. Ibn Sina's book on drugs for cardiovascular diseases. Int J Cardiol 2010;145:223.
[105] Tekol Y. The medieval physician Avicenna used an herbal calcium channel blocker, Taxus baccata L. Phytother Res 2007;21:701-2.
[106] Eknoyan G. A history of diabetes mellitus—a disease of the kidneys that became a kidney disease. J Nephrol 2006;19(Suppl 10):S71-4.
[107] The history of diabetes. URL www.med.uni-giessen.de/itr/history/diabhis.html.
[108] Majeed A. How Islam changed medicine. BMJ 2005;331:1486-7.
[109] West JB. Ibn al-Nafis, the pulmonary circulation, and the Islamic Golden age. J Appl Physiol 1985;105(6):1877-80.
[110] Siahpoosh M, Ebadiani M, Shah Hosseini G, Isafhani M, Nasrabadi AN, Dadgostar H. Avicenna the first to describe diseases which may be prevented by exercise. Iran J Public Health 2012;41(11):98-101.
[111] Osler W. Suggested scheme for the restoration of the Tomb of Avicenna. Proc R Soc Med 1914;7(Sect Hist Med):280.
[112] O'sullivan PM. The Canon Medicinae of Avicenna. Bull Med Libr Assoc 1928;17(3):14-5.
[113] Lichtwardt HA. Avicenna—philosopher and genius, teacher and surgeon. J Mich State Med Soc 1950;49(5):568-72.
[114] Weaver AD. Avicenna, 980-1037. Works in the library of the New York Academy of Medicine. Bull NY Acad Med 1955;31(4):334.
[115] Huard P. Avicenne (980-1037); Abou Ali al-Housayn ibn-Abdoullah ibn-Sina. Concours Med 1956;78(50):5357-63. [French].
[116] Galdston I. Avicenna and Islamic science. Bull NY Acad Med 1955; 31(4): 300-1.
[117] Levy R. Avicenna—his life and times. Med Hist 1957;1(3):249-61.
[118] Kuprilanov VV. Outstanding contribution of the works of Avicenna to the history of anatomy (on the occasion of the 1,000th anniversary of the birth of Avicenna). Arkh Anat Gistol Embriol 1980;79(9):109-11. [Russian].
[119] Mannan AA, Kahvic M. Ibn Sina: a tribute. Gulf J Oncolog 2010;(7):60-3.
[120] Shamsi M, Haghverdi F, Changizi Ashtiyani S. A brief review of Rhazes, Avicenna, and Jorjani's views on diagnosis of diseases through urine examination. Iran J Kidney Dis 2014;8(4):278-85.
[121] Bittar EE. A study of Ibn Nafis. Bull Hist med 1955;29:352-68.
[122] Coppola ED. The discovery of the pulmonary circulation: a new approach. Bull Hist Med 1957;31:44-77.

[123] Masic I, Dilic M, Solakovic E, Rustemepasic N, Ridjanovic Z. Why historians of medicine called Ibn al-Nafis the second Avicenna? Med Arh 2008;62(4):244-9.
[124] Masic I. On the occasion of 800th anniversary of birth of Ibn al-Nafis—discoverer of cardiac and pulmonary circulation. Med Arh 2010;64(5):309-13.
[125] Akmal M, Zulkifle M, Ansari A. Ibn Nafis—a forgotten genius in the discovery of pulmonary blood circulation. Heart Views 2010;11(1):26-30.
[126] Rodin FH. Moses Maimonides: Great physician, scientist, and philosopher. Cal West Med 1936;44(3):192-6.
[127] Barr SE. Moses Maimonides. N Engl J Med 154;250(18):779-80.
[128] Rosner F. Nephrology and urinalysis in the writings of Moses Maimonides. Am J Kidney Dis 1994;24:222-7.
[129] Gesundheit B. Maimonides' appreciation for medicine. Rambam Maimonides Med J 2011;2(1):e0018. doi: 10.5041/RMMJ.10018.
[130] Connor H. Moses Maimonides (1135-1204). J Med Biogr 2009;17(1):13. doi: 10.1258/jmb.2008.008005.
[131] Cantwell JD. On camel rides and Moses Maimonides. Proc (Bayl Univ Med Cent). 2015;28(3):406-8.
[132] Rosner F, Muntner S. Moses Maimonides' aphorisms regarding analysis of urine. Ann Intern Med 1969;71(1):217-20.
[133] Massry SG. Maimonides: physician and nephrologist. Am J Neprhol 1994;14(4-6):307-12.
[134] Kaltenstadler W. Life is short, art is long: Medical works of Moses Maimonides. Dtsch Med Wochenschr 2010;135(51-52):2563-6. [German].
[135] Rosner F, Muntner S, eds. The medical aphorisms of Moses Maimonides. NewvYork: Yeshiva Universtiy Press, 1971.
[136] Eknoyan G. On the contributions of Paracelsius to nephrology. Nephrol Dial Transplant 1996;11:1138-94.
[137] Medvei VC. The 16th century and the Renaissance. In: Medvei VC, ed. The history of clinical endocrinology: A comprehensive account of endocrinology from earliest times to the present day. New York: Parthenon Publishing, 1993:55-6,97.
[138] Morley H. The life of Girolamo Cardano of Milan, Physician 2 volumes. London: Chapman Hall, 1854.
[139] Ongaro G. Girolamo Cardano and Andreas Vesalius. Riv Stor Med 1969;13(1):51-61. [Italian].
[140] Regöly-Mérei G. The life and scientific activity of Girolamo Cardano. Orv Hetil 1971;112(38):2291-3. [Hungarian].
[141] Simili A. The figure and work of Girolamo Cardano. Riv Stor Med 1970;14(1):3-18. [Italian].
[142] Scarani P. Out of control: the life of Gerolamo Cardano (1501-1576). Pathologica 2001;93(5):565-74. [Italian].
[143] Antonello A, Calo L, Bonfante L, Mennella G, Abaterusso C, Spinello M, et al. Giovanni Battista Morgagni, a pioneer of clinical nephrology. Am J Nephrol 1999;19:222-5.
[144] Fischer WJ. Thomas Sydenham, the English Hippocrates: (1624-1689). Can Med Assoc J 1913;3(11):931-46.

[145] No Authors listed. Thomas Sydenham (1624-1689). Can Med Assoc J 1924;14(10):983-4.
[146] Bloch H. Thomas Sydenham, MD (1624-1689): the father of clinical observation. J Fam Pract 1994;38(1):80-1.
[147] Low G. Thomas Sydenham: the English Hippocrates. Aust NZ J Surg 1999;69(4):258-62.
[148] Anstey P. The creation of the English Hippocrates. Med Hist 2011;55(4):457-78.
[149] Hamid A, Mohd A, Tanzeel A, Naghma C. Diabetes mellitus from antiquity to present scenario and contribution of Greco-Arab physicians. JISHIM 2006;5:46-50.
[150] Willis T. Pharmaceutice rationalis or an exercitation of the operations in humane bodies. London: Dring Harper Leigh, 1678.
[151] Willis T. Founders of modern medicine. I Thomas Willis, MA, MD (1621-1675). Med Library Hist J 1903;1(4):264-70.
[152] van Gijn J, Gijselhart JP. Willis and his circle. Ned Tijdschr Geneeskd 2012;156(12):A4653. [Dutch].
[153] Feindel W. Thomas Willis (1621-1675)-The founder of neurology. Can Med Assoc J 1962;87(6):289-96.
[154] Ahmed AM. History of diabetes mellitus. Saudi Med J 2002;23(4):373-8.
[155] Stylianou C, Kelnar C. The introduction of successful treatment of diabetes mellitus with insulin. J R Soc Med 2009;102(7):298-303.
[156] Allan FN. The writings of Thomas Willis, MD; Diabetes 300 years ago. Diabetes 1953;2(1):74-7.
[157] Greydanus DE, Hofmann AD. Psychological factors in diabetes mellitus. Am J Dis Child 1979;133:1061-6.
[158] Bosmia AN, Tubbs RI, Clapp DC, Batzdorf U, Loukas M, Tubbs RS. Johann Conrad Brunner (1653-1727) and the first description of syringomyelia. Child Nerv Syst 2014;30(2):193-6.
[159] Keck FS, Pfeiffer EF. The first experimental diabetes mellitus. Acta Diabetol Lat 1989;26(1):79-81.
[160] Brunner JC. Experimenta nova circa pancreas, accedit diatribe de lympha et gemino pancreatis usu. Amsterdam: Apud H Wetstenium, 1683.
[161] Keck FS, Duntas LH. Brunner's missing 'Aha experience' delayed progress in diabetes research by 200 years. Hormones (Athens) 2007;6(3):251-4.
[162] Dobson M. Experiments and observations on the urine in diabetes. In: Medical Observations and Inquiries. Volume 5. London: T Cadell, 1776:298-316.
[163] Williamson RT. English physicians of the past. Newcastle: Andrew Reid, 1923:47-52.
[164] Polonsky KS. The past 200 years in diabetes. N Engl J Med 2012;367:1332-40.
[165] Furdell EL. Fatal thirst. Diabetes in Britain until insulin. Leiden, Netherlands: Brill, 2009:81-92.
[166] Sanders LJ. From Thebes to Toronto and the 21st century: an incredible journey. Diabetes Spectrum 2002;15(1):56-60.
[167] Kerr CE, Milne I, Kaptchuk TJ. William Cullen and a missing mind-body link in the early history of placebos. J R Soc Med 2008;101(2):89-92.

[168] Cawley TA. Singular case of diabetes, consisting entirely in the quality of urine; with an inquiry into the different theories of that disease. London Med J 1788;9:286-308.
[169] Longo LD. Classic pages in obstetrics and gynecology: an account of a particular change of structure in the human ovarium. Matthew Baillie, 1789. Am J Obstet Gynecol 1975;123(7):770.
[170] Young RH. The history of British gynaecological pathology. Histopathology. 2009;54(2):144-55.
[171] Somebody. The introduction of successful treatment of diabetes mellitus with insulin. R Soc Med 2009;102(7):298-303.
[172] Baillie M. The morbid anatomy of some of the most important parts of the human body, 2nd ed. London: J Johnvson, 1797.
[173] Rollo J. Causes of the diabetes mellitus, 2nd ed. London: C Dilly, 1798.
[174] Rollo J. An account of two cases of the diabetes mellitus,with remarks as they arose during the progress of the cure. London: C Dilly, 1797.
[175] Lemay P. Michel Eugene Chevreul (1786-1889). J Chem Educ 1948;25(2):62.
[176] Bourgougnon A. Michel Eugéne Chevreul. 1786-1889. J Am Chem Soc 1989;11(5):71-79.
[177] Chevreul ME. Note sur le sucre de diabetes. Ann Chim 1815;95:319-20.
[178] Fehling H. Die quantitative Bestimmung von Zucker und Stärkmehl mittelst Kupfervitriol. Ann Chemie Pharmacie 1849;72(1):106-13.
[179] Elliotson J. The principles and practice of medicine. London: J Butler, 1839.
[180] Ridgway ES. John Elliotson (1791-1868): a bitter enemy of legitimate medicine? Part II: The mesmeric scandal and later years. J Med Biogr 1994;2:1-7.
[181] Todd EM. An itinerant mermerist. Anaesth Intensive Care 2012;40(Suppl 1):5-9.
[182] Wittke G. Claude Bernard (1813-1878)-remarks on his methodology. Berl Munch Tierarztl Wochenschr 1994;107(2):37-42. [German]
[183] Jörgens V, Grüsser M. Happy birthday, Claude Bernard. Diabetes 2013;62(7):2181-2.
[184] Bernard C. Introduction ? l'étude de la Médecine Expérimentale. Paris: J-B Bailliére, 1865.
[185] Bernard C. De l'origine du sucre dans l'?conomie animale. Arch Gen Med 1848;18:303-319. [French].
[186] Foster M. Claude Bernard: a lecture. BMJ 1878;1(903):559-60.
[187] Rodriquez de Romo AC, Borgstein J Claude Bernard and fat emulsion (or the Sleeping Beauty 150 years later). Gac Med Mex 2000;136():379-86. [Spanish]
[188] Han KW. The formation and background of Claude Bernard's general physiology. Uisahak 2010;19(2):507-52. [Korean].
[189] Noble D. Claude Benard, the first systems biologist, and the future of physiology. Exp Physiol 2008;93(1):16-26.
[190] Bernard C. Mémoire sur le pancréas et sur le rôle du suc pancréatique dans les phénomènes digestifs, particulièrement dans la digestion des matières grasses neutres. Comptes rendus hebdomadaires de l'Académie des sciences 1856;1:379–563.

[191] Friedman A. Fluid and electrolyte therapy: a primer. Pediatr Nephrol 2010;25(5):843-6.
[192] Harrison HE, Darrow DC, Yannet H. The total electrolyte content of animals and its probable relation to the distribution of body water. J Biol Chem 1936;113:515-29.
[193] Gamble JL. Chemical anatomy, physiology and pathology of extracellular fluid: a lecture syllabus. Boston, MA: Harvard University Press, 1947.
[194] Granger A, Kushner JA. Cellular origins of beta cell regeneration: a legacy view of historical controversies. J Intern Med 2009;266(4):326-38.
[195] Rosenfeld L. William Prout: early 19th century physician-chemist. Clin Chem 2003;49(4):699-705.
[196] Prout W. On the nature and treatment of stomach and renal diseases, 5th ed. London: Churchill, 1848.
[197] Brock WH. The life and work of William Prout. Med Hist 1965;9:101-26.
[198] No authors listed. William Prout (1785-1850) analytical chemist. JAMA 1968;206(5):1079-80.
[199] Copeman WS. William Prout, M.D., FRS. Physician and chemist (1785- 850). Notes Rec R Soc Lond 1970;24:273-80.
[200] No authors listed. William Prout (1785-1859). Nutrition classics: Philosophical Transactions of the Royal Society of London. For the year MDCCCXXVII. Part I. Volume CXVII:355-388, 1827. XXIII. On the ultimate composition of simple alimentary substances; with some preliminary remarks on the analysis of organized bodies in general. By William Prout. Nutr Rev 1975;33(4):112-4.
[201] Ahrens R. William Prout (1785-1850): a biographical sketch. J Nutr 1977; 107(1):17-23.
[202] Nwaneri C. Diabetes mellitus: a complete ancient and modern historical perspective. WebmedCentral Diabetes 2015;6(2):WMC004831.
[203] Kark RM. A propect of Richard Bright on the centenary of his death, December 16, 1958. Am J Nephrol 1958;6:819-24.
[204] Dock W. Proteinuria: the story of 280 years of trials, errors, and rectifications. Bull NY Acad Med 1974;50:659-66.
[205] Bright R. Reports of medical cases. Selected with a view of illustrating the symptoms and cure of diseases by a reference to morbid anatomy. London: Longman Rees Orme Brown Green, 1827.
[206] Weller RO, Nester B. Historical reassessment of three kidneys originally described by Richard Bright in 1827-36. BMJ 1972;2(5816):761-3.
[207] Dunea G. History of nephrology: the middle period. Hektoen Internat: J Med Humanities. URL: http://www.hektoeninternational.org/HON-beginnings.html.
[208] MacKenzie JC. Dr. Richard Bright—a man of many parts. His bicentenary year—1789-1858. Bristol Med Chir J 1989;104(3):63-7.
[209] Mukhin NA. Richard Bright and the nephrological theory of E.M. Tareev. Klin Med (Mosk) 1990;68(1):4-7. [Russian].
[210] Young RH. Dr. Richard Bright—father of medical renal disease. Arch Pathol Lab Med 2009;133(9):136.
[211] Apollinaire B. De la Glycosurie ou diabète sucré, son traitement hygénigue. Paris: Libraire Germer Bailliére, 1883.

[212] Bouchardat A. Nouveau mémoire sur la glycosurie. Comptes rendus des séances de l'Académie des sciences 1845;20:1020.
[213] Chast F. Apollinaire Bouchardat, pharmacist, nutritionist. Ann Pharm Fr 2000;58(6 Suppl):435-42. [French].
[214] Chast F, Slama G. Apollinaire Bouchardat and diabetes. Hist Sci Med 2007;41(3):287-301. [French].
[215] Trépardoux F, Ségal A. Bouchardat and hygienic medicine. Hist Sci Med 2007;41(3):279-86. [French].
[216] Karamanou M, Koutsilieris M, Laios K, Marineli F, Androutsos G. Apollinaire Bouchardat (1806-1886): founder of modern diabetology. Hormones (Athens) 2014;13(2):296-300.
[217] Lancereaux E. Note et réflexions sur deux cas de diabéte sucrè avec alteration du pancrèas. Bull Acad Med 1877;6:1215.
[218] Lancereaux E. Le diabéte maigre: ses symptomes, son évolution, son prognostic et son traitment; ses rapports avec les altérations du pancréas. Etude comparative du diabéte maigre et du diabéte gras. In: Delahaye A, Lecrosnier E, eds. Lecons de Clinique Médicale: Paris: 1883:5–16.
[219] Peumery JJ. Étienne Lancereaux (1829-1910) sa vie, son oeuvre, ses découvertes scientifiques. Hist Sci Med 1989;23(4):279-84.
[220] Lestradet H. The 75th anniversary of the discovery of insulin. Diabetes Metab 1997;23(1):112-7. [French].
[221] Leickert KH. Insulin precursors—a historical synopsis. First diabetes treatment trials using pancreatic extracts. Arzneimittelforschung 1975;25(3):439-42. [German].
[222] Wolf G. Friedrich Theodor von Frerichs (1819-1885) and Bright's disease. Am J Nephrol 2002;22(5-6):596-602.
[223] No authors listed. Friedrich Theodor von Frerichs (1819-1885). JAMA 1963;186:511-2.
[224] Martini GA. Friedrich Theodor von Frerichs (1819-1885). Clinical picture of acute liver atrophy. Internist (Berl) 1969;10(3):74-8.
[225] Schwarz U, Ritz E. Glomerulonephritis and progression----Friedrich Theodor von Frerichs, a forgotten pioneer. Nephrol Dial Transplant 1997;12:2776-8.
[226] Thormann J, Steinberg H. Friedrich Theodor von Frerichs (1819-1885). J Neurol 2014;261(1):248-9.
[227] Young P, Finn BC, Bruetman JE, Buzzi A, Zylberman M. The outstanding achievements of Adolf Kussmaul. Rev Med Chil 2012;140(4):538-44. [Spanish].
[228] Hoffmann KF. Memories of the clinician Adolf Kussmaul (1822-1902); special reference to hydrotherapy. Hippokrates 1952;23(15):419-20.
[229] No authors listed. Adolf Kussmaul (1822-1902) – country doctor to clinical professor. JAMA 1964:189:54-9.
[230] Nogaller AM. Adolf Kussmaul (1822-1902) as a doctor, scientist, teacher. Klin Med (Mosk) 1999;77(6):63-4. [Russian].
[231] Johnson SK, Naidu RK, Ostopowicz RC, Kumar DR, Bhupathi S, Mazza JJ, et al. Adolf Kussmaul: distinguished clinician and medical pioneer. Clin Med Res 2009;7(3):107-12.

[232] Kussmaul A. Zur Lehre vom Bailliere. Uber eine eigenthumliche to desart bei Diabetischen, Uber Acetonamie. Glycerin-behandlung des Diabetes und Einspritzungen von Diastase ins blit bei dieser Kranicheit. Deutsche Arch Klin Med1874;14:1-46. [German]
[233] Breathnach CS, Westphal W. Adolf Kussmaul (1822-1902): from youth to maturity under the influence of Virchow. J Med Biogr 2003;11(1):55-61.
[234] Noyes HD. Retinitis in glycosuria. Trans Am Ophthalmol Soc 1869;4: 71-5.
[235] Kalantzis G, Angelou M, Poulakou-Rebelako E. Diabetic retinopathy: An historical assessment. Hormones 2006;5(1):71-4.
[236] Nettleship E. On oedema or cystic disease of the retinal. Roy Ophthal Lond Hosp Rep 1872;VII:343-41.
[237] Mackenzie S, Nettleship E. A case of glycosuric retinitis. Roy Ophth Lond Hosp Rep 1877;9:134.
[238] Lawford JB. British masters of ophthalmology series: Edward Nettleship FRS, FRCS (1845-1913) Br J Ophthalmol 1923;7:nil4-9. doi: 10.1136/bjo.7.1.nil4.
[239] Wolfensberger TJ, Hamilton AM. Diabetic retinopathy—an historical review. Semin Ophthalmol 2001;16(1):2-7.
[240] Naunyn B. Der diabetes mellitus. Wien: Alfred Holder, 1898.
[241] Brogard JM, Vetter T, Blickle JF. Discovery of pancreatic diabetes in Strasbourgh. Diabet Metab 1992;18(2):104-14.
[242] Caldwell J. Drug metabolism and pharmacogenetics: the British contribution to fields of international significance. Br J Pharmacol 2006;147(Suppl 1):S89-S99.
[243] Barach JH. Paul Langerhans, 1847-1888. Diabetes 1952;1(5):411-3.
[244] Campbell WR. Paul Langerhans, 1847-1888. Can Med Assoc J 1958;79(10):855-6.
[245] Becker V. 100 hundred years after Paul Langerhans' doctoral thesis on the cells of the pancreas. Dtsch Med Wochenschr 1970;95(7):358-62. [German].
[246] Wolff G, Schadenwaldt H. 1877-1977: Bibliographic annotations on Paul Langerhans—the islands were his destiny. Med Welt 1977;28(1):1-7. [German].
[247] Ebling FJG. Homage to Paul Langerhans. J Invest Dermatol 1980;75:3-5.
[248] Sakula A. Paul Langerhans (1847-1888): a centenary tribute. J R Soc Med 1988;81(7):414-5.
[249] Jollies S. Paul Langerhans. J Clin Pathol 2002;55(4):243.
[250] Langerhans P. Beiträge zur mikroscopischen anatomie der bauchspeichel druse. Dissertation. Berlin: Gustav Lange, 1869. [German].
[251] Morrison H. Contributions to the microscopic anatomy of the pancreas by Paul Langerhans (Berlin, 1869). Reprint of the German original with an English translation and an introductory essay. Bull Inst Hist Med 1937;5:259-97.
[252] Fossati P. Edouard Laguesse at Lille in 1893 created the term "endocrine" and opened the endocrinology era. Hist Sci Med 2004;38(4):433-9. [French].
[253] Laguesse E. Sur la formation des ilots de Langerhans dans le pancreas. Comptes Rendus Hebdomadaires des Seances et Memoires de la Societe de Biologie 1893;5:819–820. [French].
[254] Laguesse E. Recherches sur l'histogénie du pancreas chez le mouton. J Anat Physiol 1895;31:475–500.

[255] Laguesse E. Sur la formation des ilots de Langerhans dans le pancreas. Comptes Rendus Hebdomadaires des Seances et Memoires de la Societe de Biologie 1893;5:819–20.
[256] Debeyre A. How insulin was discovered; corollary on the scientific research of the Dijon physician Gustave-Edouard Laguesse, former professor emeritus of the Lille Univeristy Medical faculty. Prog Med (Paris) 1956;84(23):442.
[257] Goet JP. Gustave Edouard Laguesse; his demonstration of the significance of the islands of Langerhans. Diabetes 1953;2(4):322-4.
[258] Dickinson WH. Diabetes. Disease of the kidney. London: Longsmans Green, 1875.
[259] von Mering JV, Minkowski O. Diabetes mellitus nach pankreasextirpation. Zbl Klin Med 1889;10:393-4. [German]
[260] Von Mering JV, Minkowski O. Diabetes mellitus nach pankreasexstirpation. Arch Pathol Pharmak 1889-1890;26:371-87. [German].
[261] Minkowski O. Die Lehre vom pancreas. Diabetes in ihrer geschichtlichen Entwicklung. Munch Med Wschr 1929;76:311-5. [Germna].
[262] No authors listed. Oskar Minkowski (1858-1931): designer of experimental diabetes. JAMA 1967;199:754-5.
[263] Kaiser W, Völker A. Oscar Minkowski (1858-1931). Z Gesamte Inn Med 1981;36(24):973-9. [German].
[264] Jörgens V. Oscar Minkowski (1858-1931): An outstanding master of diabetes research. Hormones (Athens) 2006;5(4):310-1.
[265] Brogard JM, Blickle JF. History of the rhenish and alsacian contributions to the understanding of diabetes. Hist Sci Med 2004;38(4):421-32. [French].
[266] Dittrich HM, Hahn Von Dorshe H. The anatomical and histological investigation of the pancreas in the 19th century and till the discovery of insulin (1921). The discovery of the pancreas-diabetes by von Mering and Minkowski (1889). Anat Anz 1978;143(5):509-17.
[267] Savona-Ventura C. The history of diabetes aellitus. A Maltese perspective. Malta: Self Publication, 2002. URL: http://staff.wm.edu.mt/csav1/books/diabetes_hist.pdf.
[268] Kidd JG. Eugene Lindsay Opie, MD, 1873-1971. Am J Pathol 1971;65(3):483-92.
[269] Olcott CT. Introductory remarks on the presentation of the twenty-first Middleton Goldsmith lecture. Bull Y Acad Med 1955;31(4):275-9.
[270] Menon S, Rajesh G, Balakrishman V. Pancreas and diabetes mellitus: The relationship between the organ and the disease. J Assoc Phys India 2015;63:).1-5.
[271] Opie EL. Ssobolew and insulin. Can Med Assoc J 1952;67(5):482.
[272] Opie EL. Pathological changes affecting the islands of Langerhans of the pancreas. J Boston Soc Med Soc 1900;4(10):251-60.
[273] Opie EL. On the relationship of chronic interstitial pancreatitis to the islands of Langerhans and to diabetes mellitus. J Exp Med 1901;5(4):397-428.
[274] Opie EL. Diabetes mellitus associated with hyaline degeneration of the islands of Langerhans of the pancreas. Johns Hopkins Hosp Bull 1901;12(125):263 .
[275] Rous P. An inquiriy into certain aspects of Eugene L Opie. Arch Path 1942;34:1-6.
[276] Hughes J. Eugene L. Opie. Diabetes 1958;7(6):496-9.
[277] Hirsch JG. Eugene L. Opie, 1873-1971. Trans Assoc Am Physicians 1971;84:31-4.

[278] Ssobolew LW. Zur normalen und pathologishen Morphologie der inneren Secretion der Bauchspeicheldruse. Arch Pathol Anatomie Physiol Klin Med 1902; 168:91–128. [German].
[279] Granger A, Kushne JA. Ceulluar origins of cell regeneration: a legacy view of historical controversies. J Intern Med 2009;266(4):325-338. doi: 10.1111/j.1365-2796.2009.02156.x.
[280] Schulze W. Die Bedeutung der Langerhansschen Inseln im Paukreas. Arch Mikr Anat 1900;56:491–504. [German].
[281] Bayliss WM, Starling EH. The mechanism of pancreatic secretion. J Physiol 1902;28(5):325-53.
[282] Henriksen JH. Earnest Henry Starling (1866-1927): the scientist and the man. J Med Biogr 2005;13(1):22-30.
[283] Henriksen JH, Schaffalitzky de Muckadell OB. Secretin—the first hormone. Ugeskr Laeger 2002;164(3):320-5. [Danish].
[284] Scott RV, Tan TM, Bloom SR. Can Bayliss and Starling gut hormones cure a worldwide pandemic? J Physiol 2014;592(1):5153-67.
[285] Zuelzer GL. Über versuche einer specifischen fermentherapie des diabetes. Zeitshrift Exp Pathol Ther 1908;5:307-18. [German].
[286] Mellinghoff KH. Georg Ludwig Zuelzer's contribution to the research on pancreatic extracts. Med Welt 1972;23(16):622-6. [German].
[287] Saudek CD. 2002 Presidential address: A tide in the affairs of medicine. Diabetes Care 2003;26(2):520-5.
[288] Bliss M. The discovery of insulin. Chicago, IL: Univ Chicago, 1982.
[289] Banting FG. Diabetes and insulin. Can Med Assoc J 1926;26(3):221-31.
[290] Lane MA. The cytological characters of the areas of Langerhans. Am J Anat 1907;7:409–22.
[291] Bensley RR. Studies on the pancreas of the guinea pig. Am J Anat 1911;12:297–388.
[292] Gupta V, Garg K, Raheja S, Choudhry R, Tuli A. The histogenesis of islets in the human fetal pancreas. J Anat Soc India 2002;51(1):23-6.
[293] Granger A, Kushner JA. Cellular origins of beta cell regeneration: a legacy view of historical controversies. J Intern Med 2009;266(4):325-38.
[294] Ferner H. The insular alpha and beta cells as the source of the antagonistic principles glucagon and insulin. Mikroskopie 1951;6(1–2):1–8.
[295] No authors listed. Sir Edward Sharpey-Schafer, FRS, LLD, MD, DSc, FRCPEd. BMJ 1935;1(3874):741-2.
[296] Schafer GMS. Sir Edward Sharpey-Schafer. BMJ 1935;1:801.
[297] Writer D. Resuscitation great. Sir Edward Sharpey-Schafer and his simple and efficient method of performing artificial respiration. Resuscitation 2004;61(2):113-6.
[298] Sykes AH. Edward Schafer (1850-1935) and artificial respiration. J Med Biogr 2006;14(3):155-62.
[299] No authors listed. Old age the the vices. Russell L Cecil. J Am Geriatrics Soc 1953;1:604.
[300] Textbook Titan. MD Magazine 1958;March:78-9.
[301] In sedication to Dr. Cecil". Arthritis Rheuma 1963;6:vii-viii.
[302] In memoriam. Walsh McDermott (plus brief vita). Arthritis Rheuma 1965;8:577-80.

[303] McDermott W. Russell Lafayette Cecil. Trans Am Clin Climatol Assoc 1966;77:xlvi-xlvii.
[304] Cecil RL. On hypertrophy and regeneration of the islands of Langerhans. J Exp Med 1911;14(5):500-19.
[305] Cecil RL, Vaughan HF. Results of prophylactic vaccination against pneumonia at Camp Wheeler. J Exper Med 1919;29:457–83.
[306] Cecil RL, Larsen NP. Clinical and bacteriologic study of one thousand cases of lobar pneumonia. JAMA 1922;79:343–9.
[307] Cecil RL, Sutliff WD. The treatment of lobar pneumonia with concentrated anti-pneumococcus serum. JAMA 1928;91:2036–40.
[308] Cecil RL, Plummer N. Pneumococcus Type 1 pneumonia: a study of eleven hundred and sixty-one cases, with especial reference to specific therapy. JAMA 1931;95:1547–53.
[309] Neuhauser D, Diaz M, Chalmers I. A puzzling omission in a gret medical textbook edited by a pioneer of controlled trials. J R Soc Med 2008;101(7):381-383.
[310] Cecil RL. Textbook of medicine. Philadelphia, PA: WB Saunders, 1927.
[311] Goldman L, Schafer AI, eds. Goldman-Cecil medicine, 25th ed. Philadelphia, PA: Elsevier, 2016.
[312] Scott EL. The relation of pancreatic extract to the sugar in the blood. Proc Soc exp Med Biol 1913;10:101-3.
[313] Boehm R, Hoffmann FA. Beiträge zur Kentniss des Kohlehydratsoff- wechsels. Arch Exp Pathol Pharmakol 1878;8:295-304. [German].
[314] Macleod JJR. Studies in experimental glycosuria: I. On the existence of afferent and efferent nerve fibers, controlling the amount of sugar in the blood. Am J Physiol 1907;19:388-406.
[315] Drinker CK. Walter Bradford Cannon 1871-1945. Science 1945; 102(2654):470-2.
[316] Iaroshevskiĭ MG. Chesnokova SA. Centenary of the birth of Walter Bradford Cannon (1871-1945). Fiziol Zh SSSR Im I M Sechenova 1971;57(10):1559-62. [Russian].
[317] Joaquin Izquierdo J. Walter Bradford Cannon (1871-1945). His human general personality. In memoriam. Gac Med Mex 1972;104(1):73-6. [Spanish].
[318] Gorisch E, Gorisch R. Walter Bradford Cannon (1871-1945). The professional activities of an outstanding physiologist. Z Gesamte Hyg 1990;36(7):368-70. [German].
[319] Cooper SJ. From Claude Bernard to Walter Cannon. Emergence of the concept of homeostatis. Appetite 2008;51(3):419-27.
[320] Cannon WB, Shohl AT, Wright WS. Emotional glucosuria. Am J Physiol 1911;29:280-7.
[321] Cannon WB. The secretion of the adrenal glands during emotional excitement. Science 1911;2:907.
[322] Henderson Y, Underhill FP. Acapnia and glycosuria. Am J Physiol 1911; 28:275-89.
[323] Knox WE. Sir Archibald E Garrod. Genetics 1967;56(1):1-6.
[324] Dronamraju K. Profiles in genetics: Archibald E. Garrod (1857-1936). Am J Hum Genet 1992;51(1):216-9.
[325] Garrod AE. Lettsomian lectures on glycosuria. Lancet 1912;1:480-8.

[326] Folin O, Denis W, Smillie WG. Some observations on "emotional glycosuria" in man. J Biol Chem 1914;17:519-20.
[327] Allen FM. Studies concerning glycosuria and diabetes, Cambridge, MA: Harvard University Press, 1913.
[328] Allen FM, Stillman E, Fitz R. Total dietary regulation in the treatment of diabetes. New York: Rockefeller Institute Medical Research, Monograph 11, 1919.
[329] Duncan GG. Frederick Madison Allen 1879-1964. Diabetes 1964;13:318-9.
[330] No authors listed. Frederick Madison Allen 1879-1964. Metabolism 1964;13:383-5.
[331] Grott JW, Swiezawska E. Frederick Madison Allen (1879-1964) and his contributions to the knowledge of diabetes mellitus. Pol Tyg Lek 1965;20(49):1872. [Polish].
[332] Mazur A. Why were "starvation diets" promoted for diabetes in the pre-insulin period? Nutr J 2011;10:23. doi: 10.1186/1475-2891-10-23.
[333] Westman EC, Yancy WS Jr., Humphreys M. Dietary treatment of diabetes mellitus in the pre-insulin era (1914-1922). Perspect Biol Med 2006;49(1):77-83.
[334] Barnett DM. Elliot Proctor Joslin. American National Biography. New York: Oxford Press, 1999:282–83.
[335] Joslin EP. The obligation and the opportunity of the chiropodist in the treatment of diabetes. J Am Podiatr Med Assoc 2007;97(4):271-3.
[336] Joslin EP. Influence of bile on metabolism. J Boston Soc Med Sci 1899;3(10):259-63.
[337] Joslin EP. Present day treatment and prognosis in diabetes. Am J Med Sci 1915;150:485-96.
[338] Beaser RS, Campbell A. The Joslin guide to diabetes. Boston, MA: Joslin Diabetic Center, 2016.
[339] Kleiner IS, Meltzer SJ. Retention in the circulation of dextrose in normal and depancreatized animsl and the effects of an intravension injection of an emulsion of pancreas upon this retention. Proc Nat Acad Sc 1915;1:338-40.
[340] Kleiner IS. The actions of the intravenous injections of pancreatic emulsions in experimental diabetes. J Biochem 1919;40:153-70.
[341] Kleiner IS. The action of intravenous injections of pancreas emulsions in experimental diabetes. Am J Physiol 1919;29:306-10.
[342] Barthold SW. Unsung heroes in the battle against diabetes. ILAR J 2004;45(3):227-30.
[343] Tattersal R. Pancreatic organotherapy for diabetes, 1889-1921. Med Hist 1995;39(3):288-316.
[344] James T. History of medicine. Paulesco. S Afr Med J 1992;82(2):123-5.
[345] Dominguez LJ, Licata G. The discovery of insulin: what really happened 80 years ago. Ann Ital Med Int 2001;16(3):155-62. [Italian].
[346] Laron Z. Nicolae C. Paulescu—scientist and politician. Isr Med Assoc J 2008;10(7):491-3.
[347] Paulesco NC. Action de l'extrait pancreatique injecte dans le sang, chez un animal diabetique. Comptes Rendus des Seances de la Societe de Biologie 1921;85:555–9. [French].

[348] D Haulica I. Professor Nicolae C. Paulesc-the true discoverer of insulin. Rev Med Chir Soc Med Nat Iasi 2001;105(3):602-5. [Romanian].
[349] Roth J, Qureshi S, Whitford I, Vranic M, Kahn CR, Fantus IG, et al. Insulin's discovery: new insights on its ninetieth birthday. Diabetes Metab Res Rev 2012;28(4):293-304.
[350] Bliss M. The eclipse and rehabilitation of JJR Macleod, Scotland's insulin laureate. J R Coll Physicians Edinb 2013;43(4):366-73.
[351] Pavel I, Sdrobici D. N. Paulescu, discoverer of insulin. 50th anniversary of the discovery of that hormone. Med Interna (Bucur) 1972;24(11):1285-94. [Romanian].
[352] Kenéz J. Who invented insulin? (Charles H. Best, Frederick Grant Banting). Orv Hetil 1978;119(44):2693-9. [Hungarian]
[353] No authors listed. Frederick Grant Banting (1891-1941), codiscovered of insulin. JAMA 1966;198(6):660-1.
[354] Raju TN. A mysterious something: the discovery of insulin and the 1923 Nobel Prize for Frederick G Banting (1891-1941) and John JR Macleod (1876-1935). Acta Paediatr 2006;95(10):1155-6.
[355] Berche P, Lefrère JJ. The return to life with insulin. Ann Endocrinol (Paris) 2010;71(4):243-8. [French]
[356] De Herder WW. Heroes in endocrinology: Nobel Prizes. Endocr Connect 2014;3(3):R94-R104.
[357] Pai-Dhungat JV, Parikh F. Frederick Banting (1891-1941). J Assoc Physicians India 2015;63(3):114.
[358] Barron M. The relation of the islets of Langerhans to diabetes with special reference to cases of pancreatic lithiasis. Surg Gynec Obstet 1920;31:437–448.
[359] Hobart A, Reimann MD. Moses Barron and Banting. JAMA 1967;199(1):48.
[360] Shampo MA, Kyle RA. Charles Best—codiscoverer of insulin. Mayo Clin Proc 2004;79(12):1546.
[361] Macleod J. Insulin and diabetes. BMJ 1922;2:833.
[362] Macleod JJR: History of the researches leading to the discovery of insulin (1922), letter of Macleod to Col. Albert Gooderham. Bull History Med 1978;52:295-312.
[363] Shampo MA, Kyle RA. Macleod John J.R.--Nobel prize for discovery of insulin. Mayo Clin Proc 2006;81(8):1006.
[364] Banting FG, Best CH. Pancreatic extracts. J Lab Clin Med 1922;7:464–72.
[365] Banting FG, Best CH, Collip JB, Campbell WR, Fletcher AA. Pancreatic extracts in the treatment of diabetes mellitus. Preliminary report. Can Med Assoc J 1922;12:141–146.
[366] Noble RL. Memories of James Bertram Collip. Can Med Assoc J 1965; 93(26):1356-1364.
[367] Barr ML, Rossiter RJ. James Bertram Collip 1892-1965. Biogr Mem Fellows R Soc 1973;19:234.
[368] Bangham DR. H.H. Dale and the London Centre for WHO standards—some milestones of the early years. Dev Biol Stand 1999;100:11-5.
[369] Harvey AM. Pharmacology's giant: John Jacob Abel. Johns Hopkins Med J Suppl 1974;135(4):245-58.

[370] Murnaghan JH, Talalay P. John Jacob Abel and the crystallization of insulin. Perspect Biol Med 1967;10(3):334-80.
[371] Himsworth HP. Diabetes mellitus: its differentiation into insulin-sensitive and insulin-insensitive types. Diabet Med 2011;28(12):1440-4. (Reprinted from Management of diabetes mellitus, BMJ 1936).
[372] Black D, Gray J. Sir Harold Percival Himsworth, K.C.B.-19 May 1905—1 November 1993. Biogr Mem Fellows R Soc 1995;41:199-218.
[373] Himsworth R. Sir Harold Himsworth. Diabet Med 2011;28(11):1438-9.
[374] Krentz AJ, Hitman GA. Sir Harold Himsworth and insulin insensitivity 75 years on. Diabet Med 2011;28(12):1435.
[375] Sanger F. The free amino groups of insulin. Biochem J 1945;39(5):507-15.
[376] Sanger F, Thompson EO, Kitai R. The amide groups of insulin. Biochem J 1955;59(3):509-18.
[377] Sanger F. Chemistry of insulin: determination of the structure of insulin opens the way to greater understanding of life processes. Science 1959;129(3359):1340-4.
[378] Deckert T. Hans Christian Hagedorn (1888-1971). Ugeskr Laeger 2007;169(35):2883. [Danish].
[379] Poulsen JE. Hans Christian Hagedorn (1888-1971. Dan Medicinhist Årbog 1978;9-45. [Danish].
[380] Kruse PR. The hospital pharmacies in Copenhagen and their professional importance. Dan Medicinhist Årbog 2005;33:163-70. [Danish].
[381] Philipson LH, Bell G, Polonsky KS. Donald F. Steiner MD, 1930-2014: Discoverer of proinsulin. PNAS (Proc Nat Acad Sci) 2015;112(4):940-1.
[382] Frandsen CS, Dejgaard TF, Madsbad S. non-insulin drugs to treat hyperglycaemia in type 1 diabetes mellitus. Lancet Diabetes Endocrinol 2016 Mar 8. pii: S2213-8587(16)00039-5.
[383] Kooti W, Farokhipour M, Asadzadeh Z, Ashtary-Larky D, Asadi-Samani M. The role of medicinal plants in the treatment of diabetes; a systematic review. Electron Physician 2016;8(1):1832-42.
[384] Röder PV, Wu B, Liu Y, Han W. Pancreatic regulation of glucose homeostasis. Exp Mol Med 2016;48:e219.
[385] Salas-Salvado J, Guasch-Ferré M, Lee CH, Estruch R, Clish CB, Ros E. Protective effects of the Mediterranean diet on type 2 diabetes and metabolic syndrome. J Nutr 2016 Mar 9. pii:jn218487.
[386] Voormolen DN, Abell SK, James R, Hague WM, Mol BW. Diagnostic criteria and treatment for gestational diabetes mellitus. Semin Reprod Med 2016;34(2):102-9.
[387] Luczynski W, Glowinska-Olszewska B, Bossowski A. The influence of clinical and genetic factors on the development of obesity in children with type 1 diabetes. Diabetes Metab Res Rev 2016 Mar 6. doi: 10.1002/dmrr.2797.
[388] Backes JM, Kostoff MD, Gibson CA, Ruisinger JF. Statin-assocviated diabetes mellitus: review and clinical guide. South Med J 2016;109(3):167-73.
[389] Brunström M, Carlberg G. Effect of antihypertensive treatment at different blood pressure levels in patients with diabetes mellitus: systematic review and meta-analyses. BMJ 2016 Feb 24;352:i717. doi: 10.1136/bmj.i717.

[390] Knip M, Siljander H. The role of the intestinal microbiota in type 1 diabetes mellitus. Nat Rev Endocrinol 2016;12(3):154-67.
[391] Clements JN, Bello L. Insulin glargine 300 units/mL: a new basal insulin product for diabetes mellitus. Am J Health Syst Pharm 2016;73(6):359-66.
[392] Barnosky A, Shah L, Meah F, Emanuele N, Emanuele MA, Mazhari A. A primer on concentrated insuins: what an internist should know. Postgrad Med 2016 Feb 27.
[393] Dholakia S, Mittal S, Quiroga I, Gilbert J, Sharples E, Pleog RF et al. Pancreas transplantation: past, present, future. Am J Med 2016 Mar 7. pii; S0002-9343(16)30199-1.
[394] Jewett EA, Anderson MR, Gilchrist GS. The pediatric subspecialty workforce: public policy and forces for change. Pediatrics 2005;116(5):1192-202.
[395] Pierce JS, Kozikowski C, Lee JM, Wysocki T. Type 1 diabetes in very young children: a model of parent and child influences on management and outcomes. Pediatr Diabetes 2015 Dec 29. doi: 10.1111/pedi.12351.
[396] Kim SH. Maturity-onset diabetes of the young: what do clinicians need to know? Diabetes Metab J 2015;39(6):468-77.
[397] Greydanus DE. Endocrine disorders. In: Hofman AD, ed. Adolescent medicine. Menlo Park, CA: Addison-Wesley, 1983:160-80.
[398] Greydanus DE, Hofmann AD. Endocrine disorders. In: Hofman AD, Greydanus DE, eds. Adolescent medicine, 2nd ed. Norwalk, CT: Appleton Lange, 1989:231-56.
[399] Greydanus DE. Exercise and insulin-requiring diabetes mellitus. In: Luckstead EF, Greydanus DE, eds. Medical care of the adolescent athlete. Los Angeles, CA: Professional Medical Information, 1993:177-8.
[400] Greydanus DE. Endocrine disorders. In: Hofman AD, Greydanus DE, ds. Adolescent medicine, 3rd ed. Norwalk, CT: Appleton Lange, 1997:314-47.

SECTION TWO: ACKNOWLEDGMENTS

Chapter 3

About the Authors

Donald E. Greydanus, MD, Dr. HC (Athens), FAAP, FSAM (Emeritus), FIAP (HON) is Professor and Founding Chair of the Department of Pediatric and Adolescent Medicine, as well as Pediatrics Program Director at the Western Michigan University Homer Stryker MD School of Medicine (WMED), Kalamazoo, Michigan, USA. He is also Professor of Pediatrics and Human Development at Michigan State University College of Human Medicine (East Lansing, Michigan, USA) as well as Clinical Professor of Pediatrics at MSU College of Osteopathic Medicine in East Lansing, Michigan, USA. Received the 1995 American Academy of Pediatrics' Adele D. Hofmann Award for "Distinquished Contributions in Adolescent Health", the 2000 Mayo Clinic Pediatrics Honored Alumnus Award for "National Contributions to the field of Pediatrics," and the 2003 William B Weil, Jr., MD Endowed Distinguished Pediatric Faculty Award from Michigan State University College of Medicine for "National and international recognition as well as exemplary scholarship in pediatrics." Received the 2004 Charles R Drew School of Medicine (Los Angeles, CA) Stellar Award for contributions to pediatric resident education and awarded an honorary membership in the Indian Academy of Pediatrics—an honor granted to only a few pediatricians outside of India. Was the 2007-2010 Visiting Professor of Pediatrics at Athens University, Athens, Greece and received the Michigan State University College of Human Medicine Outstanding Community Faculty Award in 2008. In 2010 he received the title of Doctor Honoris Causa from the University of Athens (Greece) as a "distinguished scientist who through outstanding work has bestowed praise and credit on the field of adolescent medicine (Ephebiatrics)." In 2010 he received the Outstanding Achievement in

Adolescent Medicine Award from the Society for Adolescent Medicine "as a leading force in the field of adolescent medicine and health." In 2014 he was selected by the American Medical Association as AMA nominee for the ACGME Pediatrics Residency Review Committee (RRC) in Chicago, Illinois, USA. Past Chair of the National Conference and Exhibition Planning Group (Committee on Scientific Meetings) of the American Academy of Pediatrics and member of the Pediatric Academic Societies' (SPR/PAS) Planning Committee (1998 to Present). In 2011 elected to The Alpha Omega Alpha Honor Society (Faculty member) at Michigan State University College of Human Medicine, East Lansing, Michigan. Former member of the Appeals Committee for the Pediatrics' Residency Review Committee (RRC) of the Accreditation Council for Graduate Medical Education (Chicago, IL) in both adolescent medicine and general pediatrics. Numerous publications in adolescent health and lectureships in many countries on adolescent health. E-mail: donald.greydanus@med.wmich.edu

Joav Merrick, MD, MMedSci, DMSc, born and educated in Denmark is professor of pediatrics, child health and human development, Division of Pediatrics, Hadassah Hebrew University Medical Center, Mt Scopus Campus, Jerusalem, Israel and Kentucky Children's Hospital, University of Kentucky, Lexington, Kentucky United States and professor of public health at the Center for Healthy Development, School of Public Health, Georgia State University, Atlanta, United States, the medical director of the Health Services, Division for Intellectual and Developmental Disabilities, Ministry of Social Affairs and Social Services, Jerusalem, the founder and director of the National Institute of Child Health and Human Development in Israel. Numerous publications in the field of pediatrics, child health and human development, rehabilitation, intellectual disability, disability, health, welfare, abuse, advocacy, quality of life and prevention. Received the Peter Sabroe Child Award for outstanding work on behalf of Danish Children in 1985 and the International LEGO-Prize ("The Children's Nobel Prize") for an extraordinary contribution towards improvement in child welfare and well-being in 1987. E-mail: jmerrick@zahav.net.il

Chapter 4

About the Department of Pediatric and Adolescent Medicine, Western Michigan University Homer Stryker MD School of Medicine (WMED), Kalamazoo, Michigan, USA

Mission and Service

The Western Michigan University Homer Stryker MD School of Medicine was started in 2012 and its first class of medical students began in 2014. The Department of Pediatric and Adolescent Medicine has a pediatric residency program which is accredited by the Accreditation Council for Graduate Medical Education (ACGME) in Chicago, Illinois, USA and the current residency program in Pediatrics started in 1990.

The WMED Department of Pediatric and Adolescent Medicine has a commitment to a comprehensive approach to the health and development of the child, adolescent, and the family. The Department has a blend of academic general pediatricians and pediatric specialists. Our Pediatric Clinic team provides a broad spectrum of general well and sick child care (birth through 18 years) including immunizations, monitoring general physical and emotional growth, motor skill development, sports medicine (including participation evaluations and evaluation of common sports injuries), child abuse evaluations, and psychosocial or behavioral assessment. WMED Pediatrics believes in immunizations as a protection against preventative disease processes. Our Pediatrics Clinic is undergoing a transformation to a patient-centered medical home (PCMH). A patient-centered medical home is a way to deliver coordinated and comprehensive primary care to our infants, children, adolescents and young adults. It is a partnership between individuals and families within a health care setting, which allows for a more efficient use of resources and time to improve the quality of outcomes for all involved through care provided by a continuity care team.

Research activities

The Department has a variety of research projects in adolescent medicine, neurobehavioral pediatrics, adolescent gynecology, pediatric diabetes mellitus, asthma, and cystic fibrosis. The WMED Department of Pediatric and Adolescent Medicine has published a number of medical textbooks: Essential adolescent medicine (McGraw-Hill Medical Publishers), The pediatric diagnostic examination (McGraw-Hill), Pediatric and adolescent psychopharmacology (Cambridge University Press), Behavioral pediatrics, 2nd edition (iUniverse Publishers in New York and Lincoln, Nebraska), Behavioral pediatrics 3rd edition (New York: Nova Biomedical Books); 4th Edition: In press. Pediatric practice: Sports medicine (McGraw-Hill), Handbook of clinical pediatrics (Singapore: World Scientific), Neuro-developmental disabilities: Clinical care for children and young adults (Dordrecht: Springer), Adolescent medicine: Pharmacotherapeutics in medical disorders (Berlin/Boston: De Gruyter), Adolescent medicine: Pharmacotherapeutics in general, mental, and sexual health (Berlin/Boston: De Gruyter), Pediatric psychodermatology (Berlin/Boston: De Gruyter), Substance abuse in adolescents and young adults: A manual for pediatric and primary care clinicians (Berlin/Boston: De Gruyter), and tropical pediatrics (New York: Nova); Second edition in press.

The Department has edited a number of journal issues published by Elsevier Publishers covering pulmonology (State of the Art Reviews: Adolescent Medicine—AM:STARS), genetic disorders in adolescents (AM:STARS), neurologic/neurodevelopmental disorders (AM:STARS), behavioral pediatrics (Pediatric Clinics of North America), pediatric psychopharmacology in the 21st century (Pediatric Clinic of North America), nephrologic disorders in adolescents (AM:STARS), college health (Pediatric Clinics of North America), adolescent medicine (Primary Care: Clinics in

Office Practice), behavioral pediatrics in children and adolescents (Primary Care: Clinics in Office Practice), adolescents and sports (Pediatric Clinics of North America), and developmental disabilities (Pediatric Clinics of North America). The Department has also edited a journal issue on musculoskeletal disorders in children and adolescents for the American Academy of Pediatrics' AM:STARs; in April of 2013 a Subspecialty Update issue was published in AM:STARs.

The department has developed academic ties with a variety of international medical centers and organizations, including the Queen Elizabeth Hospital in Hong Kong, Indian Academy of Pediatrics (New Delhi, India), the University of Athens Children's Hospital (First and Second Departments of Paediatrics) in Athens, Greece and the National Institute of Child Health and Human Development in Jerusalem, Israel.

Contacts

Professor Dilip R Patel, MD, current chair and Professor Donald E Greydanus, MD, founding chair, Department of Pediatric and Adolescent Medicine
Western Michigan University Homer Stryker MD School of Medicine
1000 Oakland Drive, D48G, Kalamazoo, MI 49008-1284, United States
E-mail: dilip.Patel@med.wmich.edu
and Donald.greydanus@med.wmich.edu
Website: http://www.med.wmich.edu

Chapter 5

About the National Institute of Child Health and Human Development in Israel

The National Institute of Child Health and Human Development (NICHD) in Israel was established in 1998 as a virtual institute under the auspices of the Medical Director, Ministry of Social Affairs and Social Services in order to function as the research arm for the Office of the Medical Director. In 1998 the National Council for Child Health and Pediatrics, Ministry of Health and in 1999 the Director General and Deputy Director General of the Ministry of Health endorsed the establishment of the NICHD.

Mission

The mission of a National Institute for Child Health and Human Development in Israel is to provide an academic focal point for the scholarly interdisciplinary study of child life, health, public health, welfare, disability, rehabilitation, intellectual disability and related aspects of human development. This mission includes research, teaching, clinical work, information and public service activities in the field of child health and human development.

Service and Academic Activities

Over the years many activities became focused in the south of Israel due to collaboration with various professionals at the Faculty of Health Sciences (FOHS) at the Ben Gurion University of the Negev (BGU). Since 2000 an affiliation with the Zusman Child Development Center at the Pediatric Division of Soroka University Medical Center has resulted in collaboration around the establishment of the Down Syndrome Clinic at that center. In 2002 a full course on "Disability" was established at the Recanati School for Allied Professions in the Community, FOHS, BGU and in 2005 collaboration was started with the Primary Care Unit of the faculty and disability became part of the master of public health course on "Children and society". In the academic year 2005-2006 a one semester course on "Aging with disability" was started as part of the master of science program in gerontology in our collaboration with the Center for Multidisciplinary Research in Aging. In 2010 collaborations with the Division of Pediatrics, Hadassah Hebrew University Medical Center, Jerusalem, Israel around the National Down Syndrome Center and teaching students and residents about intellectual and developmental disabilities as part of their training at this campus.

Research Activities

The affiliated staff have over the years published work from projects and research activities in this national and international collaboration. In the year 2000 the International Journal of Adolescent Medicine and Health and in 2005 the International Journal on Disability and Human Development of De Gruyter Publishing House (Berlin and New York) were affiliated with the National Institute of Child Health and Human Development. From 2008 also the International Journal of Child Health and Human Development (Nova Science, New York), the International Journal of Child and Adolescent Health (Nova Science) and the Journal of Pain Management (Nova Science) affiliated and from 2009 the International Public Health Journal (Nova Science) and Journal of Alternative Medicine Research (Nova Science). All peer-reviewed international journals.

NATIONAL COLLABORATIONS

Nationally the NICHD works in collaboration with the Faculty of Health Sciences, Ben Gurion University of the Negev; Department of Physical Therapy, Sackler School of Medicine, Tel Aviv University; Autism Center, Assaf HaRofeh Medical Center; National Rett and PKU Centers at Chaim Sheba Medical Center, Tel HaShomer; Department of Physiotherapy, Haifa University; Department of Education, Bar Ilan University, Ramat Gan, Faculty of Social Sciences and Health Sciences; College of Judea and Samaria in Ariel and in 2011 affiliation with Center for Pediatric Chronic Diseases and National Center for Down Syndrome, Department of Pediatrics, Hadassah Hebrew University Medical Center, Mount Scopus Campus, Jerusalem.

INTERNATIONAL COLLABORATIONS

Internationally with the Department of Disability and Human Development, College of Applied Health Sciences, University of Illinois at Chicago; Strong Center for Developmental Disabilities, Golisano Children's Hospital at Strong, University of Rochester School of Medicine and Dentistry, New York; Centre on Intellectual Disabilities, University of Albany, New York; Centre for Chronic Disease Prevention and Control, Health Canada, Ottawa; Chandler Medical Center and Children's Hospital, Kentucky Children's Hospital, Section of Adolescent Medicine, University of Kentucky, Lexington; Chronic Disease Prevention and Control Research Center, Baylor College of Medicine, Houston, Texas; Division of Neuroscience, Department of Psychiatry, Columbia University, New York; Institute for the Study of Disadvantage and Disability, Atlanta; Center for Autism and Related Disorders, Department Psychiatry, Children's Hospital Boston, Boston; Department of Pediatric and Adolescent Medicine, Western Michigan University Homer Stryker MD School of Medicine, Kalamazoo, Michigan, United States; Department of Paediatrics, Child Health and Adolescent Medicine, Children's Hospital at Westmead, Westmead, Australia; International Centre for the Study of Occupational and Mental Health, Düsseldorf, Germany; Centre for Advanced Studies in Nursing, Department of General Practice and Primary Care, University of Aberdeen, Aberdeen, United Kingdom; Quality of Life Research Center, Copenhagen, Denmark; Nordic School of Public Health, Gottenburg, Sweden, Scandinavian Institute of Quality of Working Life, Oslo, Norway;

The Department of Applied Social Sciences (APSS) of The Hong Kong Polytechnic University Hong Kong.

TARGETS

Our focus is on research, international collaborations, clinical work, teaching and policy in health, disability and human development and to establish the NICHD as a permanent institute in Israel in order to conduct model research and together with the four university schools of public health/medicine in Israel establish a national master and doctoral program in disability and human development at the institute to secure the next generation of professionals working in this often non-prestigious/low-status field of work.

Contact

Joav Merrick, MD, MMedSci, DMSc
Professor of Pediatrics
Medical Director, Health Services,
Division for Intellectual and Developmental Disabilities,
Ministry of Social Affairs and Social Services,
POB 1260, IL-91012 Jerusalem, Israel.
E-mail: jmerrick@zahav.net.il

Chapter 6

About the Book Series "Public Health: Practices, Methods and Policies"

Public health is a book series with publications from a multidisciplinary group of researchers, practitioners and clinicians for an international professional forum interested in the broad spectrum of public health issues. Books already published:

- Rubin IL, Merrick J, eds. Environment and public health: Environmental health, law and international perspectives. New York: Nova Science, 2014.
- Shek DTL, Siu AMH, Merrick J, eds. Tomorrow's leaders: Service leadership and holistic development in Chinese university students. New York: Nova Science, 2015.
- Siziya S, Mazaba ML, Merrick J, eds. Arbovirus: Public health experience from Zambia. New York: Nova Science, 2015.
- Obeng C, Obeng SG, Merrick J, eds. Health issues in diverse cultures. New York: Nova Science, 2015.
- Friedman BD, Merrick J, eds. Public health, social work and health inequalities. New York: Nova Science, 2015.
- Rubin IL, Merrick J, eds. Environmental health disparities: Costs and benefits of breaking the cycle. New York: Nova Science, 2016.
- *Mazaba ML, Siziya S, Merrick J, eds. Smoking and adolescence: International public health experiences. New York: Nova Science, 2016.*

- Merrick J, ed. Public health: Some international perspectives. New York: Nova Science, 2016.
- Greydanus DE, Merrick J. Medical history: Some perspectives. New York: Nova Science, 2016.
- Rubin IL, Merrick J, eds. Public health: International aspects on environment and health. New York: Nova Science, 2016.
- Shek DTL, Ma C, Lin L, Merrick J, eds. Education in Hong Kong: Service leadership for university students. New York: Nova Science, 2016.
- Shek DTL, Siu AMH, Leung H, Merrick J, eds. Higher education in Hong Kong: Nurturing students to be caring service leaders. New York: Nova Science, 2016.
- Marufu T, Siziya S, Mazaba ML, Merrick J, eds. Measles: Epidemiology and control of measles in the Gweru urban district in Zimbabwe. New York: Nova Science, 2016.
- Hegamin-Younger C, Merrick J, eds. Caribbean adolescents: Misuse and abuse of alcohol. New York: Nova Science, 2016.

Contact

Professor Joav Merrick, MD, MMedSci, DMSc
Medical Director, Health Services
Division for Intellectual and Developmental Disabilities
Ministry of Social Affairs and Social Services
PO Box 1260, IL-91012 Jerusalem, Israel
E-mail: jmerrick@zahav.net.il

SECTION THREE: INDEX

INDEX

D

E

F

G

H